SECRETS OF PILATES

SECRETS OF
PILATES

SALLY SEARLE &
CATHY MEEUS

IVY PRESS

This edition published in the UK in 2017 by
Ivy Press
Ovest House
58 West Street
Brighton
BN1 2RA
www.quartoknows.com

First published in 2001

British Library Cataloguing-in-Publication Data
A catalogue record for this book is available from the British Library

ISBN: 978-1-78240-465-1

This book was conceived, designed and produced by
Ivy Press
Art Director: Peter Bridgewater
Publisher: Sophie Collins
Editorial Director: Steve Luck
Designers: Kevin Knight, Jane Lanaway and Ginny Zeal
Project Editor: April McCroskie
Picture Research: Vanessa Fletcher
Photographer: Calvey Taylor-Haw
Illustrations: Sarah Young, Coral Mula and Michael Courtney
Three-dimensional models: Mark Jamieson
Editorial Assistant: Jenny Campbell

Printed in China

10 9 8 7 6 5 4 3 2 1

Note from the publisher
Although every effort has been made to ensure that the information
presented in this book is correct, the authors and publisher cannot
be held responsible for any injuries which may arise.

Beneficial
People of all ages will benefit from a well-rounded Pilates exercise program.

HOW TO USE THIS BOOK

This book comprises five chapters. The first introduces Joseph Pilates, charts the history of the development of his exercise methods, and examines why they are suitable for people of all ages. Chapter two gives all the information you will need before embarking on an exercise program. Chapter three prepares you for the practical bodywork by explaining the basics and outlining a suggested routine. Chapter four takes a look at foundation exercises, offering in-depth explanations and step-by-step guidelines. When you have mastered this section and are confident with the foundation exercises you will be ready for the final chapter, which takes a look at more advanced progression exercises.

Further Information

While the information presented within the pages of this book is useful to anyone considering taking lessons in Pilates exercise, it is important to understand that it is not a substitute for instruction from a qualified Pilates teacher.

This book is for reference purposes only, and ideally the exercises within it should be carried out under the supervision of a trained professional. Please see page 219 for some useful addresses to help guide you.

Background
The first chapter of the book looks at the basic principles of Pilates.

Planning

Easy-to-follow tables outline suggested exercise routines that you can follow on a daily basis.

Exercises

Each exercise is described in detail with step-by-step instructions to show you how to carry it out effectively.

Alignment

Supine alignment

The body, in particular the spine, is at its most relaxed when lying down on the back in what is called the supine position. It is therefore best to begin your posture adjustment in this position. For this introduction to the Pilates routine, it is helpful to have someone to observe and correct you. Obviously, if you are in a class, your teacher will do this for you. If you are exercising at home, persuade a family member or friend to help you. Brief them on the key features that you are trying to achieve and ask them to let you know when you have got it right.

Key alignment points

Lie down on a padded surface, supporting your head with a flat pillow or folded towel if necessary. Working from feet to head, check the following:
• Your feet and knees are hip-width apart, facing forward, and parallel.
• Your hips are level.
• Your arms are resting a short distance from your sides, palms may be up or down, elbows are slightly bent.
• Your shoulders are level and relaxing away from your ears.
• Your neck is lengthened.
• Your head is not tilted forward nor back.

Neutral pelvis

Viewed from the side the pelvis should be held in a way that maintains the normal concave curve of the lower back at the waist—the lumbar curve. If the pelvis tips forward, the lumbar curve is exaggerated; if it tips back, the curve is flattened. Either of these positions can create back strain if it forms part of your habitual posture. The exact position of neutral pelvis is different for each individual. Locating the neutral position for your pelvis in the supine position (see below) will be among your first tasks.

Analysis

Black-and-white pages analyze each exercise and give tips on how to gain maximum benefits from your exercise program.

Getting it straight
The first lesson of Pilates is learning how to position yourself correctly.

Each time you commence an exercise session, it is important to establish a well-aligned posture. At first you may need to make many adjustments, but your body will eventually learn these new habits of alignment.

Introduction

Mind & body in harmony
*The Pilates system of exercise provides
unrivaled integration of mind and body.*

If you are seeking a balanced
approach to toning your body,
correcting alignment, and improving
your posture and coordination, then
Pilates is the perfect exercise system
for you to follow.

Mind & body

Modern fitness programs increasingly
recognize the strong link between the
mind and body. Physical practices to
develop a healthy, fit body also encourage
psychological and emotional well-being.
Conversely, effective mental relaxation
and meditational techniques help to dispel
the damaging physical consequences
of stress and depression.

The exercise system devised by Joseph
Pilates acknowledges and builds on this
link between mind and body. The aim of
his exercises is to use mental focus to gain
a deeper understanding of your body
and develop its potential for the benefit
of your overall health and well-being. The
emphasis is on developing your mental
awareness of how your body moves—an
insight that many of us have lost. This is
perhaps best described as bringing your
mind into your body, rather than using
your mind to gain control over your body.

One of the differences between the
Pilates approach and that of many other
exercise systems is in the precision of the
individual movements that make up each
exercise. Newcomers to Pilates often
wonder how such tiny movements can
bring such enormous benefits. But as you
become more familiar with the exercises,
it will become apparent that the system
is so effective precisely because the
movements are so carefully focused.

A personal journey

Embarking on a Pilates-style exercise
program can be seen as a first step on
the path to a new physique and perhaps

even a new approach to life. Pilates recognizes that every individual has their own capabilities and potential and encourages you to proceed at your own pace. Your developing confidence with each exercise will be your indicator of progress, rather than any arbitrary timescale or other external measure. This book aims to give the newcomer to Pilates an introduction to the principles of this exercise system.

Working with a Teacher

You can achieve a lot by practicing the fundamentals on your own, but to progress you need the guidance of a qualified Pilates teacher. It is hoped that this book will inspire you to join a class and make Pilates exercise a regular part of your life.

THE PILATES SYSTEM

Pilates is devised to bring your body back into healthy alignment and to teach new postural habits so that you can move freely without strain. The exercises strengthen the body from its "center" to provide the stability from which harmonious and stress-free movement of the limbs can derive. It is important to note that the exercises need to be carried out precisely according to the instructions and therefore demand full mental engagement. This first chapter explains the background and principles underlying the Pilates system and provides useful anatomical information to help you understand how your body works and what happens to it when you exercise.

Joseph Pilates: The Man & His Work

Strong & supple

By following the exercise program devised by Joseph Pilates you can achieve a strong, supple body.

Joseph Hubertus Pilates was born in Düsseldorf, Germany, in 1880. As a child he suffered from asthma and rickets and this early experience of ill-health shaped his attitude toward the importance of physical fitness throughout his life. In his youth he made determined efforts to build and strengthen his body. He became an all-round athlete and also began to develop the system of body-conditioning exercises that he later termed "Contrology."

At the outbreak of World War I he was in England teaching self-defense to British detectives. However, he was interned along with his fellow countrymen for the duration of the war and during this period he used his system of exercises to keep himself and the other internees fit and healthy.

After the war ended Pilates returned to his native Germany. During the early 1920s he began to work with some of the best-known dancers of the day. Then in 1926 he emigrated to the United States, where he founded his first exercise studio. By the 1940s his unique exercise regime had built up a growing reputation as a beneficial counterbalance to the sometimes damaging demands of dance training and he built up a wide clientele among New York's community of dancers and actors. Since then, many world-famous show business personalities have benefited from the Pilates Method of exercise. In recent years many sports stars have also found Pilates exercises valuable for redressing the physical imbalances imposed by rigorous sports training.

The Pilates legacy

In the decades between the founding of the Pilates Studio and the death of Joseph Pilates in 1967, numerous students became proficient and knowledgeable in his methods. Some of these students, including Ron Fletcher and Eve Gentry, went on to found their own Pilates-style exercise studios and there are now many different strands of Pilates teaching. Inevitably, each teacher gives their own emphasis and interpretation to the basic exercise program that was laid down by its founder. Those who are interested in the authentic voice of Joseph Pilates himself can refer to his books, *Your Health* (1934) and *Return to Life Through Contrology* (1945).

PILATES PHYSIQUE

A Pilates-trained body is immediately recognizable for its symmetry and toned appearance. Key features of such a body include: a lengthened spine, in which the natural curves are neither flattened nor exaggerated; level shoulders that are free from any tendency to hunch toward the ears; the appearance of a long neck; a firm abdomen, without any bulging of the diaphragm; graceful, free-moving limbs; level hips; and strong, but not overmuscled, legs. Body movements flow smoothly and without effort from such a physique.

Key features

The distinguishing characteristics of a Pilates-trained body may start to become noticeable within a few months of starting regular Pilates practice. The progress you make will depend on your body type and the amount of time you are able to devote to your practice.

Graceful, strong limbs

long neck

Lengthened
spine

Level hips

Firm
abdomen

The Principles

Inspiration from the ancients
*Pilates based much of his thinking on ancient
ideas of physical perfection.*

In devising his own system of exercises Joseph Pilates drew on physical training systems from many different philosophical and cultural traditions. He was particularly impressed by the writings of the early Greeks, but was also absorbed by various elements from Eastern thinking and even studied the movements of animals. The general principles underlying each of his exercises give testimony to the extent to which his method is intended to reach both body and mind.

Concentration & control

In Pilates the key to success is the engagement of the mind in the actions of the muscles of the body. This mental focus encourages the development of body awareness—this is a sensitivity to the effect of different movements and muscle actions on the body as a whole. To achieve it you first need to develop your ability to focus without distraction on the movements you are trying to perform in order to rediscover "forgotten" muscles and ways of moving. Only when you are concentrating in this way will you be able to gain control over your muscles and move in the way you want to, rather than being dictated to by habit.

Precision & coordination

Your aim is to perform each exercise in precisely the way described. The difference between moving correctly and incorrectly is often apparently minuscule to the newcomer to Pilates, but gaining awareness of these subtle nuances of body use is one of the key lessons you will be learning. Ultimately the aim is to be able to link series of movements in a coordinated and balanced fashion.

Fluidity & flexibility

Pilates exercises are designed to encourage smooth movements that flow from one position to the next. There should be no hurried or jerky actions; these risk straining and shortening the muscles. The increased flexibility created by regular Pilates practice enhances the movement possibilities that are available to you and the fluidity with which you can perform them.

Centering & breathing

The Pilates approach aims to help you develop strength at the center of your body, in the muscles of the torso, in order to free the movement of the limbs. To achieve this you also need to learn to breathe in a way that brings adequate oxygen into your body but that does not encourage excessive relaxation at the center during exercise.

THE PRINCIPLES AT WORK

As you start to perform the exercises described later in this book, keep reminding yourself of the principles that should underlie your approach to each movement. All the elements described on the previous page need to be brought into play in even the simplest exercise.

Fluidity & flexibility

Be aware that each movement you make is part of a larger sequence and should be performed with a sense of the overall flow. Enjoy your newfound mobility and grace as you develop.

Concentration & control

Keep bringing your focus back to the action you are performing in order to achieve control.

Centering & breathing

Maintain awareness at all times of a sense of strength and stability in your center. Check that you are inhaling and exhaling at the appropriate stage in each exercise and that your breathing technique is correct.

Precision & coordination

Fight the temptation to ignore any part of the exercise instruction or to take shortcuts. Accuracy will ensure that each element of the exercise links logically to the next.

The Key Body Structures

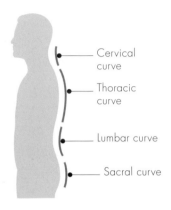

Cervical curve

Thoracic curve

Lumbar curve

Sacral curve

Natural curves
*The four curves of the back provide
natural shock-absorbing capability.*

Before embarking on a Pilates
program, it is important to learn
some basic facts about the key
anatomical features that are of particular
relevance to the exercises you will be
performing. These features will also be
mentioned from time to time during the
course of the book.

The spine
The spine is the bony column that protects
the spinal cord and also connects and
supports the entire skeleton. The spine is
made up of 33 separate bones known

as vertebrae. This segmented structure
gives the spine its flexibility and strength.
Each vertebra is joined to its neighbor
by ligaments that control its range of
movement. Intervertebral disks provide a
cushioning layer of cartilage that prevents
friction between the vertebrae.

Viewed from behind, the spine should
appear straight, but in profile it has four
natural curves. These curves lend the
spine a degree of springiness that allows
it to absorb shocks that will be incurred
during normal movement. One of the
objectives of Pilates exercise is to maintain
or reestablish this healthy profile, which
can sometimes be distorted through poor
postural habits.

The shoulders
The shoulders are the points at which
the arms are joined to the torso. Each
shoulder is a meeting point for three
separate bones: the collarbone (clavicle),
shoulder blade (scapula), and upper
arm bone (humerus). The collarbone is
connected to the top of the breastbone
(sternum). The relative position of the
shoulders is a vital determinant of the
body's overall posture.

The pelvis

The pelvis is the bony basin that contains the body's lower abdominal organs. It is joined to the lower part of the spine and provides the attachment points for the legs—the hip joints. The vertical muscles of the abdomen (see page 22) are attached to the lower part of the pelvis—the pubic bone. Proper alignment of the pelvis is a key factor in maintaining the stability of the torso and is a major priority in all Pilates exercises.

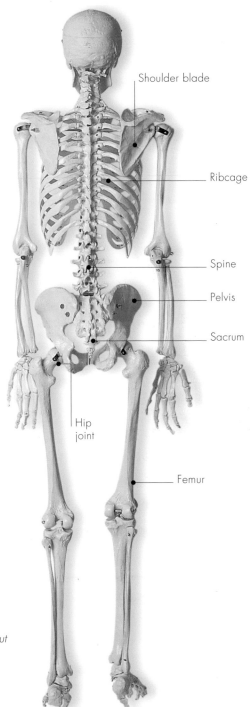

Shoulder blade

Ribcage

Spine

Pelvis

Sacrum

Hip joint

Femur

Strengthening

Many medical experts believe that Pilates increases bone density throughout the body, reducing the risk of fractures and disorders, including osteoporosis.

THE MAIN MUSCLES

The muscles are contractile tissues that create movement in the body. They work in opposing pairs; when one muscle contracts, the other relaxes to allow the movement to take place. With regular use, muscles become stronger and tighter, but they also need to be stretched in order to allow flexibility in the relaxed state. If muscles are relatively unused they become weak and slack and also lose their elasticity.

Muscles

The main muscles and muscle groups mentioned in this book are illustrated here.

Deltoid

Pectorals

Biceps

External abdominal oblique

Transversus abdominus

Rectus abdominus

Quadriceps

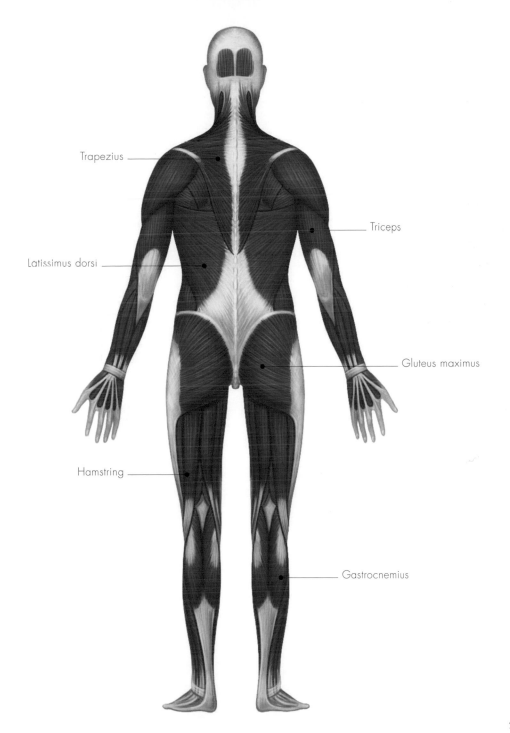

Trapezius

Triceps

Latissimus dorsi

Gluteus maximus

Hamstring

Gastrocnemius

The Girdle of Strength

A strong center

All Pilates exercises rely on the stability provided by the girdle of strength.

According to Pilates theory, all movement of the body should originate from a strong center. Joseph Pilates called this the "girdle of strength" or "powerhouse." When the torso is held in correct and stable alignment, the limbs are free to move without strain. A strong torso, in which the muscles of the abdomen and back actively support the spine and internal organs, has a graceful, energetic appearance and is less likely to suffer from strains and injuries due to poor posture. If the girdle of strength is weak, the strain of moving or maintaining position is taken on by other muscles, such as those of the legs, shoulders, and back, which are not designed for such work.

The centering muscles

One of your first tasks as a Pilates beginner is to locate and become familiar with your girdle of strength. The body has its center of gravity within the abdominal cavity just below the navel and this area should also be the stable center of the torso, from which you can move safely.

Whenever you perform a Pilates exercise you will be instructed to engage your centering muscles, except, of course, when you are specifically aiming to reach a relaxed state. This means you should tighten, without tensing, your abdominal muscles on the out-breath. To do this you should visualize your navel being drawn toward your spine ("navel to spine" is a common mantra). You also need to engage your pelvic floor (see pages 54–55), buttock muscles, and the latissimus dorsi (lats).

Maintaining muscle tone

Some forms of exercise increase muscle bulk as well as physical strength, but the effect of Pilates is to tone and lengthen the muscles, creating the possibility of a wide range of movements in a well-balanced body.

Getting into good habits

Regularly reminding yourself to engage
your centering muscles before undertaking
any kind of movement, particularly a
potentially strenuous lifting task, is a
valuable way of building the principles
of Pilates into your everyday life. If you
do nothing else in terms of regular Pilates
practice, this action alone will bring
benefits since it will protect you from injury
while you are undertaking normal tasks.
Good habits as well as bad ones can
become second nature and you will soon
find that you will be engaging your
centering muscles without conscious
effort. You will find that as you practice
engaging your girdle of strength your
body will benefit from increased stability.

STRONG CENTER IN ACTION
When you engage your centering muscles you are freeing your body to move in a safe and harmonious way. As your abdominal muscles become stronger with regular Pilates practice, you will find that you can move with increasing fluidity and ease. The illustrations here show how engaging the centering muscles will ease movement in a variety of positions.

Sitting
To achieve a correct, strain-free sitting posture you need to support your spine by engaging your centering muscles.

On all fours
To maintain a neutral spine in this position you need to engage the centering muscles, without allowing tension to restrict your breathing.

Long neck

Shoulders down

Centering muscles engaged

Neutral spine

Flexing forward

In this position the spine is extremely vulnerable unless it is supported by strongly engaged centering muscles. This is especially important if you are lifting a weight from this position.

Spine
supported
by centering
muscles

Knees flexed

Standing at ease

This apparently relaxed posture is achieved only when the muscles of the abdomen are fully engaged supporting the spine and preventing loss of alignment.

Who Benefits from Pilates?

Sport and Pilates
*Pilates exercise is a perfect
adjunct to sports training.*

Pilates has an unrivaled track record as a safe and effective method of body conditioning for people of all ages. It can also help to correct physical imbalances that have arisen from ingrained, poor postural habits.

Back pain

Many people try Pilates because they are suffering from back pain caused by postural faults. The emphasis that Pilates places on strengthening the support that the abdominal muscles give to the spine is just what back pain sufferers need.

Occupational problems

Many forms of sports or dance training focus on particular actions that are relevant to that activity, and this often leads to bodily imbalances. For example, a tennis player will use and develop muscles on the side on which he or she holds the racket. This can force the body out of alignment and strain and injury are a common consequence. Those engaged in occupations that involve repetitive movements, such as computer operators or assembly-line workers, are similarly at risk from strain. Pilates helps to prevent and correct such imbalances, and supports recovery from injury.

Joint problems

Strain on the joints is often the result of failure to engage the appropriate muscles involved in a particular action of the body. This can exacerbate chronic inflammation of the joints (arthritis) and in some cases may be a contributory cause. Pilates teaches you to use your body in way that is free from excessive strain and it strengthens key muscles that protect weight-bearing joints such as the hips and knees.

Body beautiful

Perhaps the majority of Pilates students are inspired by the prospect of developing a more streamlined figure. One of the key benefits of this form of exercise is that it tones the muscles and helps you achieve a flatter stomach, tighter buttocks, and firmer thighs. However, Pilates is not primarily a fat-burning form of exercise. If you are carrying excess body fat, your appearance will still benefit from Pilates

A Word of Warning

Be sure to read the advice on getting started on page 36 before embarking on any of the exercises in this book.

training, but if you are anxious to lose weight, you may need to make dietary adjustments and add some aerobic activity, such as regular walking, to your Pilates practice.

PILATES FOR EVERYONE
Pilates exercise is suitable for people of all ages. It has as much relevance for older people entering retirement as it does for those much younger. Provided that proper caution is observed and expert advice sought when appropriate (see page 36), you can start to exercise the Pilates way whether you are male or female, young or old, and whether you are already fit or have not exercised for many years. Some examples of categories of people who can benefit from Pilates are illustrated here.

Sports buffs
You can help to minimize sports injuries by adding Pilates exercise to your regular training.

Older people
Pilates is a low impact form of exercise that is ideal for those with health problems or who have not exercised recently.

Young people
You can learn healthy patterns of movement and build strength and flexibility that will benefit you throughout life.

New mothers

Once you are past the immediate postnatal period, Pilates exercise will help you regain tone in your abdominal muscles and pelvic floor.

Those on the mend

Pilates exercise can help you regain strength and mobility after trauma such as broken bones and muscle strains.

Pilates & Other Therapies

Manipulative therapies
Many osteopaths and chiropractors recommend Pilates exercise as an adjunct to their treatments.

The Pilates approach to exercise was revolutionary at the time when it first became widely known. However, decades later, the experience of the thousands of people who have benefited from this system worldwide provides an irrefutable testimony to the effectiveness of the exercises. Many of Pilates' ideas have now been adopted by other fitness trainers and also into mainstream physical therapy. Physicians often recommend Pilates exercise as part of a rehabilitation program following injury. With the agreement of your doctor, you can safely incorporate Pilates practice alongside most medical treatments. It is also widely recommended by osteopaths.

Similar therapies

Pilates has much in common with the Alexander Technique and the Feldenkrais Method. The founders of these systems, Frederick Matthias Alexander (1869–1955) and Moshe Pinchas Feldenkrais (1904–1984), were contemporaries of Joseph Pilates. Whether or not these bodywork pioneers knew each other personally, they drew on similar sources of inspiration. With their common emphasis on balanced body use, these exercise systems can be used together.

Body–mind therapies

Pilates was one of the first body-mind therapies to originate in the West. However, Eastern cultures have ancient traditions that recognize and build on the interaction between body and mind. Those who have practiced forms of exercise, such as yoga, may find it easier to achieve the focus required than those who have never done so. Moreover, the emphasis on stretching is also common to both practices. Yet it is important to be aware of some basic differences between these systems, notably the breathing techniques recommended. Such differences can sometimes lead to conflict if both forms of exercise are used alongside each other.

Pilates Lifestyle

Joseph Pilates had his own views on the wider aspects of health and fitness, and made recommendations on such diverse topics as diet, bodily cleanliness, and the benefits of exposure to sunshine. Many of his ideas have stood the test of time. Modern advocates of Pilates exercise do not necessarily follow all of his original recommendations. You do not have to adopt a rigid lifestyle in order to benefit from the Pilates exercise system.

PREPARING FOR PILATES

The Pilates exercises in this book are all based on matwork and therefore no specialized equipment or clothing is necessary. However, there are some important preliminaries that you will need to think about before embarking on this exercise program. This chapter outlines the essential medical precautions you should take and the self-assessment body checks that should be carried out to identify any areas of weakness or misalignment that may need to be addressed in your program.

Before You Start

Get advice
It is sensible to tell your medical practitioner if you plan to add Pilates exercise to a treatment program.

Pilates aims to restore natural and healthy ways of using your body. In this sense it is a safe and suitable form of exercise for everyone. Effective practice of Pilates exercises depend on full engagement of body and mind. Therefore, there are some basic, commonsense precautions you should take. It is always important to seek medical advice before starting any new exercise program if you have a medical condition for which you are receiving treatment. In addition, you should consult your doctor if you have not exercised regularly for several years or if you have suffered significant injury.

Pregnancy & childbirth

Avoid all Pilates exercise in the first 12 weeks of pregnancy. Some Pilates exercises are safe to do in the later stages, especially if you already have some experience of this form of exercise. But you should always seek medical advice and the guidance of a qualified Pilates teacher to help you devise a program of exercises that is suitable for pregnancy. Pilates exercise is also a great way of getting back into shape after childbirth, but consult your doctor about when it is safe to start exercising before doing so.

When not to exercise

Any condition or factor that disrupts your ability to focus will make your practice less valuable and may incur the risk of injury. Do not exercise in any of the following circumstances:
- Within two hours of a meal.
- After drinking alcohol or taking mood-altering drugs such as tranquilizers.
- You have a fever or feel unwell.
- You are in pain following an injury.
- You have been taking over-the-counter or prescribed pain-relieving medication.

During exercise

To avoid strain and to gain maximum
benefit, be careful to perform the
exercises exactly as described. Do not
exceed the number of repetitions advised,
or progress to the more difficult exercises,
until you are sure you have mastered the
basics. As you perform each exercise
it is normal to experience a stretching
sensation in certain areas or to feel
tiredness or aching in previously unused
muscles. However, at no stage should you
feel actual pain. If this occurs, discontinue
the exercise and recheck the instructions;
you may be getting something wrong.
If you are unable to find the cause of the
pain—that is, to discover any error you
may be making, exclude that exercise
from your routine until you are able to
obtain the necessary guidance from
an experienced Pilates teacher.

BODY CHARACTERISTICS

The first stage of body self-assessment is to teach yourself visual awareness of the ideal body alignment. This acts as a basis for comparison when you assess the alignment and other characteristics of your own body. The feet are the basis for our standing posture, so it is normal to check from the feet upward. Look for the ideal characteristics illustrated on this page. Remember that none of us is perfect and that most of us deviate from the ideal in at least one or two respects.

Pelvis aligned—neither hip higher than the other

Knees facing forward—neither bowed nor knock-kneed

Feet parallel facing forward

Aiming for alignment

Pilates exercise aims to help you achieve symmetrical alignment of your shoulders and hips and of your head and neck over your spine. Such symmetry is not only pleasing to look at but also provides the basis for strain-free movement.

Shoulders
level

Neck straight

Shoulders not
too far back
or forward

Healthy
back
curves

Lengthened
spine

Knees
soft

Body Checks

Positioning
*Your shoulders should be level
and your hips aligned. Your head should
be directly over your spine.*

Ideal body alignment balances the
heaviest areas of the body—head,
ribcage, and pelvis—over one another
to create maximum stability and minimum
stress on the spine. Misalignment occurs
when one of these elements shifts away
from the center—for example, if the head
pokes forward, the spine tends to angle
backward to compensate. This stresses the
muscles and ligaments of the spine, making
injury more likely. Trying to redress a
primary fault may create additional faults.

Head & neck
The head is, for its size, the heaviest part of
the body. To avoid experiencing strain its
weight should be balanced evenly over the
neck and spine, neither tipping to either
side nor being held too far forward or back.

Shoulders
The shoulders should always appear to
drop in a relaxed manner away from the
neck. They should also align horizontally
with one another. In profile the shoulders
should be held neither too far forward nor
too far back.

Curves of the back
We have already seen that the spine has
both convex and concave curves when it is
viewed in profile. These curves should not
be flattened or exaggerated in any way.

Pelvis
The position of the pelvis is critical for
good posture. In profile the pelvis should
neither tip forward excessively, which
exaggerates the curve in the lower back,
nor backwards, which over-flattens this
curve. Pilates teaches you to adopt a healthy,
neutral pelvis position (see page 48).

Knees & legs

The position of the knees is in part determined by the alignment of the hip joint. The kneecaps should face directly forward and the knee joints should not angle inward (knock knees) or outward (bow legs). In profile the upper and lower legs should be aligned vertically between hips, knees, and ankles. If the lower leg curves back away from the vertical line then the knees are said to be hyperextended.

Ankles & feet

When standing, your feet should face directly forward and carry your weight evenly across the soles of the feet.

IS THIS YOU? The photographs on these pages illustrate some common postural faults. These may develop as a result of an inherited tendency or may be due to habitual poor posture. Pilates can help correct many of these faults, although it may mitigate rather than totally eliminate some problems. If you recognize your own faults here, do not be discouraged, but use the knowledge that you have corrective work to do to act as an incentive for your Pilates practice.

Uneven shoulders

Uneven pelvis

Common faults

Many, if not most of us habitually stand in a misaligned posture. Such "relaxed" positions do not in fact provide the body with rest, but create strain that distorts and stresses the supporting structures of the back.

Head
poked
forward

Shoulders
rounded
forward

Pelvis
pushed
forward

Foot Faults

Weight on inside of feet
*This fault often accompanies a
tendency to knock knees.*

Weight on outside of feet
*This fault often accompanies a
bow-legged appearance.*

Shoulders
forced back

Clothes, Equipment & Space

Clothing for comfort
Choose clothing for your Pilates practice that allows complete freedom of movement.

When you mention Pilates, some people immediately think of expensive fitness studios containing complicated exercise machines. It is true that some forms of Pilates exercise do use specially designed equipment. But matwork, the form of Pilates exercise with which this book is concerned, is wonderfully uncluttered and is therefore ideal for practicing at home. There are, however, a few basic items that you will need in order to get the most out of your exercise sessions.

Clothes

It is a matter of common sense that you need to wear light garments, with no tight waistbands. In a class you may be encouraged to wear relatively close-fitting items, such as leotards, cycling shorts, and T-shirts. This is to allow the instructor to observe your body alignment and movements more closely. At home such considerations do not apply, although you may find it easier to judge the accuracy of your performance if you avoid large, baggy garments. Matwork exercises should be carried out without shoes.

Equipment

It is useful to have the following simple items on hand:
- A thin pillow or folded towel to provide support for the head during certain floor exercises.

- For some exercises you will need a
  long scarf or piece of fabric about
  39 inches (1 meter) long by 8 inches
  (20 centimeters) wide. If you prefer,
  you could buy an exercise band from
  a sports supplier.
- Some form of padding for the floor
  surface is advised. You may want to
  obtain an exercise mat, but you can
  easily improvise with a thick rug or
  a folded blanket.
- Eventually you may reach the stage
  where you want to use weights to
  increase the challenge of the exercises.

Space

Pilates exercise can be practiced in any
space large enough for you to lie down
with your arms outstretched. Choose a
warm but well-ventilated room with a
nonslip floor surface in a part of the
home where you will not be disturbed.

REEDUCATING BODY & MIND

You are now familiar with the principles of Pilates, so you are ready to get down to some practical work. In this chapter you will be focusing on mastering each of the basic techniques that underpin all Pilates exercises. Don't skimp on this section or you will find that your progress through the foundation exercises in the next chapter will be impaired. At the end of this chapter you will also find advice on how to plan and schedule your exercise sessions in order to achieve balanced results.

Alignment

Getting it straight
*The first lesson of Pilates is learning
how to position yourself correctly.*

Each time you commence an exercise session, it is important to establish a well-aligned posture. At first you may need to make many adjustments, but your body will eventually learn these new habits of alignment.

Supine alignment

The body, in particular the spine, is at its most relaxed when lying down on the back in what is called the supine position. It is therefore best to begin your posture adjustment in this position. For this introduction to the Pilates routine, it is helpful to have someone to observe and correct you. Obviously, if you are in a class, your teacher will do this for you. If you are exercising at home, persuade a family member or friend to help you. Brief them on the key features that you are trying to achieve and ask them to let you know when you have got it right.

Head neither
forward nor back

Shoulders away
from neck

Hips level

Key alignment points

Lie down on a padded surface, supporting
your head with a flat pillow or folded
towel if necessary. Working from feet to
head, check the following:

- Your feet and knees are hip-width apart,
  facing forward, and parallel.
- Your hips are level.
- Your arms are resting a short distance
  from your sides, palms may be up or
  down, elbows are slightly bent.
- Your shoulders are level and relaxing
  away from your neck.
- Your neck is lengthened.
- Your head is not tilted forward nor back.

Neutral pelvis

Viewed from the side the pelvis should
be held in a way that maintains the
normal concave curve of the lower
back at the waist—the lumbar curve.
If the pelvis tips forward, the lumbar
curve is exaggerated; if it tips back,
the curve is flattened. Either of these
positions can create back strain if it
forms part of your habitual posture.
The exact position of neutral pelvis is
different for each individual. Locating
the neutral position for your pelvis in
the supine position (see below) will
be among your first tasks.

Knees forward
and parallel

Feet forward
and parallel

THE NEUTRAL POSITION

On the previous pages you were instructed how to adjust your basic body alignment in the supine position. Here, you will take this further and begin to learn how to relax and enhance your awareness of your body alignment. Of particular importance is the procedure for locating the neutral position for your pelvis. This preparatory relaxation routine can be used as your regular starter exercise before performing other Pilates exercises. Some people like to play relaxation tapes during this exercise.

1 *From the basic supine position described on the previous pages, bend your knees and place your feet flat on the floor hip-width apart. Be aware of the equal distribution of weight between the center of the heel and the outer and inner parts of the ball of each foot. Feel your body relaxing into the floor, your muscles softening and your spine lengthening. Allow your spine to adopt a natural position. Visualize your shoulder blades relaxing down your back, but do not force any movement. Also relax your jaw and facial muscles.*

2 *Roll your pelvis slowly from one side to the other. Do this several times, returning to the midpoint when you have finished.*

From Above

3 *After a few moments of relaxation, tilt your pelvis forward so that your pubic bone moves downward and the hollow between your lower spine and the floor increases. Keep the rest of your body and your legs relaxed as you do this.*

Throughout all of these exercises, keep your pelvis aligned horizontally, with your feet in line with your knees and hips.

4 *Next, tilt your pelvis back by drawing your navel toward your spine and lifting the pubic bone so that the hollow in your back flattens and there is no longer any space between your lower back and the floor.*

5 *Now return to a relaxed midpoint between these two extremes, in which the pelvis is level, neither tipping forward nor back. Repeat steps 3 to 5 five times. When you are done there should be a slight gap between your lower back and the floor. This is your neutral pelvis position.*

The Pelvic Floor

Coccygeus | Levator ani

Pelvic floor muscles
*These internal muscles provide vital
support for the organs within the pelvis.*

When we refer to the centering muscles, this not only includes the familiar stomach muscles at the front of the abdomen, but it also involves the hammock of muscles that holds the internal organs within the pelvis. Although the pelvis does vary between men and women (in women it's shallower and broader) it is vital for all of us to be aware of our pelvic floor and to exercise its muscles. These muscles are among the most important of all, but many people are unaware of their existence and don't know how to bring them into active use.

Pelvic floor muscles

The pelvic floor is a mesh of muscles and ligaments that extends from the pubic bone at the front of the pelvis, passes under the pelvic opening between the legs, and joins to the base of the spine. These muscles surround and control the neck of the bladder and the urethra (outlet from the bladder), the anus, and—in women—the vagina.

Why are they important?

When they are toned and active, the pelvic floor muscles provide strong support for the pelvic organs, including the bladder, and uterus (women) or prostate (men), during physical activity. They also help to provide control of urination and defecation. If your pelvic floor muscles are slack—as a result of lack of use, obesity, or childbirth—you risk developing stress incontinence (leakage of urine when pressure within the abdomen is increased, such as during exertion or coughing). There is also a greater likelihood of prolapse of the internal organs.

In Pilates terms, the pelvic floor muscles are the lowest part of the girdle of strength that stabilizes and strengthens the torso as a whole, which is why you will be required to align them in the "neutral pelvis" position at the beginning of many

Pilates exercises. These muscles are also extremely important for initiating the toning of the postural muscles deep within the abdomen. The need for balance in your physical training dictates that all of the centering muscles are developed to the same degree, otherwise you will not achieve the harmonious results that you are seeking. For these reasons, be sure to build pelvic floor exercises into your regular exercise routine.

Not Just for Women

Many people believe that slack pelvic floor muscles are a purely female problem. This is far from the truth. Men need to maintain a firm pelvic floor as well. Many of the urinary problems that men may suffer in middle age and beyond can be ameliorated by toning the pelvic floor.

53

ENGAGING THE PELVIC FLOOR
The following exercise should be a regular part of your Pilates routine. The movement is hard to see in a photograph or when demonstrated by someone else; you really have to try it yourself and learn what it feels like. Once you have learned to recognize the sensation of tightening the pelvic floor you can practice this movement anytime, anywhere. The main technique you need to try to master is that of keeping the buttocks and abdominal muscles relaxed while you engage those of the pelvic floor—but this is always a challenge.

1 *Lie on the floor in with your knees bent and your feet on the floor (see step 1, page 50). Engage the muscles of the pelvic floor as if you were trying to stop urinating midstream. As you do this, place one hand on your buttocks to check that you have not also tightened your buttock muscles. Hold for as long you can, breathing normally throughout.*

Jaw relaxed

Shoulders relaxed

2 *In the same position, engage the pelvic floor muscles again. This time place your hand on your lower abdomen, just above the pubic bone, to check that you are not overgripping the abdominal muscles or the muscles at the front of the thighs at the same time. When you are able to isolate your pelvic floor muscles, repeat the exercise five more times, holding for a minimum of ten seconds each time.*

Knees hip-width apart

Thighs relaxed

Feet flat
on floor

Buttocks
relaxed

Engaging the Mind

Body image
Think of your body as a movable model to help you visualize the movements you should make.

One of the key characteristics of Pilates exercise is that it aims to enhance conscious control of the body. In naming his exercise system Contrology, Joseph Pilates was emphasizing the importance of this mental aspect of the exercises.

He noticed that most people carry out physical actions without any conscious direction from the brain, operating on an automatic level. Pilates perceived this as a problem that reinforces habitual movements that are harmful to posture and health. He believed the solution to

this problem was conscious control of the physical actions of the body and described the result as a "reawakening" of thousands of brain cells. This premise may not be accurate in neurological terms, but those who regularly practice the Pilates exercise method, focusing their mental engagement in the process, say they feel more alert and energetic.

The power of self-belief

One of the first mental challenges you will meet is the initial difficulty you will almost certainly encounter when trying even the simplest exercises for the first time. Coordinating your breathing technique with the correct use of particular muscles is not easy for any newcomer to Pilates.

At this early stage in your Pilates program you need to bring to bear a sense of commitment to the process of learning a new discipline and also a firm belief in your own power to improve. You must accept that enhancing your control over your body is a long-term project, but you should have confidence that it is one in which you will ultimately succeed.

Techniques for mental focus

Body awareness is a two-way street—
as well as learning to give accurate
instructions to the muscles of your body,
you also need to try to develop your
sensitivity to the sensations and messages
that they send back to your brain. To focus
effectively on the muscle actions of the
body you need to eliminate all distractions.
Apart from taking the obvious practical
steps to minimize potential outside
interruptions, such as telephone calls,
you will benefit from developing your
inner powers of concentration, too.
Many people find that their concentration
benefits enormously from practicing some
form of meditation. There are numerous
techniques that you can try, from simple
breathing meditations to more elaborate
methods. Some basic visualization
exercises are described on the
following pages.

Model motion
Visualization can aid concentration, thus helping you attain the correct body movement.

VISUALIZATIONS
In Pilates most people find that their grasp of the exercises is improved if they use visualizations to help them picture the movement they are trying to create. Each person's imagination works in a different way but the visualizations on this page are useful for most people.

Pelvic stability
To help you anchor your pelvis while performing abdominal curls and similar exercises, imagine that the area from your pubic bone to the bottom of the ribcage is set in concrete.

Lengthening
In the supine position you need to keep a sense of lengthening through the spine. Prevent tension from creeping into this action by visualizing a cord attached to the top of your head that is gently stretching your head and neck away from your body. Imagine another cord similarly pulling your tailbone toward your feet.

Curling the spine

Several exercises, including the spine lift (see pages 86–87), ask you to curl and uncurl the spine. It is important to maintain a sense of lifting as well as curling and to imagine each vertebra lifting up separately from the floor as you do this. You could visualize the process as seeing the sprockets of a gear wheel disengaging link by link from a chain.

Navel to spine

One way to picture this fundamental action is to imagine a piece of string attached to your navel running through your body and emerging from your spine at the back. When you draw your navel to your spine it is as if someone were pulling this string to bring your navel closer to your backbone.

Breathing

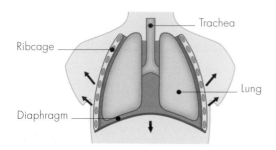

Inspiration
When you breathe in, the diaphragm flattens and the ribcage expands.

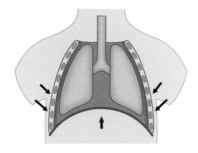

Expiration
When you breathe out, the diaphragm domes and the ribcage contracts.

When we breathe we are taking in oxygen, one of the vital ingredients that the body needs to produce energy for movement and other functions. Efficient breathing is therefore a prerequisite for optimum physical performance and it is easy to understand why Joseph Pilates emphasized the importance of breathing correctly during exercise.

Thoracic breathing

Some forms of deep breathing involve distending the abdomen as you inhale. This is not recommended in Pilates; it allows excessive relaxation of the abdominal muscles, which is not desirable during exercise because it leads to instability at your center. The breathing technique that is taught for Pilates exercise is known as thoracic or rib breathing. In this method you aim to keep your abdominals and other centering muscles engaged while your ribcage expands with the in-breath. Your shoulders should remain relaxed and should not hunch up as you inhale. On the out-breath the ribcage contracts down toward the waist and expels the waste air. During the out-breath you should be aware of all your centering muscles, including the pelvic floor, being actively engaged and drawing toward the center.

Breathing sequence

In almost every Pilates exercise you inhale before initiating a movement. Then as you begin to exhale, start the exercise. In an exercise involving more than one movement element, you may be required to pause and take an in-breath before completing the exercise on a second out-breath. Moving on the out-breath helps you to engage your centering muscles throughout the exercise and prevents any build up of unwanted tension. This breathing method also helps you avoid "doming" of the abdominals during curls (see pages 102–103), which can lead to the development of a bulging abdomen.

Body Release

To help dispel tension in the muscles and joints, lie down in the supine position (see pages 48–49) and breathe steadily. Imagine that each in-breath is drawing air into your body through the soles of your feet. As the breath moves through the legs and into the torso it softly envelops the joints and muscles, releasing any stiffness.

BREATHING EXERCISES

It is worthwhile practicing rib breathing as a separate exercise every time you do a Pilates workout until you are confident that you have thoroughly mastered the technique. It may seem strange at first to be inhaling while your lower abdomen is pulled in, but you will soon find that this way of breathing starts to come naturally. In the exercise shown here your hands should be placed on your ribcage to help heighten your awareness of the expansion and contraction of the ribcage as you breathe. Some Pilates teachers recommend wrapping a long scarf around your ribcage during breathing practice as another way of achieving this. Use whatever method works best for you but always ensure you perform this exercise in front of a mirror.

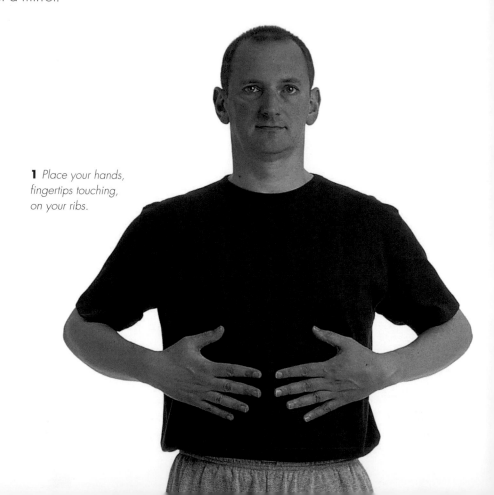

1 *Place your hands, fingertips touching, on your ribs.*

2 *Breathe in and watch hands move apart.*

Shoulders down

Ribcage expanded

Abdomen pulled in

3 *Breathe out and watch hands move close together.*

Rest & Relaxation

Kneeling rest position
This relaxation position is most useful after strenuous exercises for the back (see page 122).

Effort and relaxation are two sides of the same coin; you cannot have one without the other. If you do not use your muscles, you cannot appreciate the benefits of relaxation; if you never relax, then your muscles will not work to their optimum capacity. Because of this, every effective exercise program builds in a phase of relaxation and the Pilates method is no exception. You must set a few minutes aside for relaxation at the end of each practice, in order to allow any tension that was built up during your session to drain away. This will enable your body to assimilate the benefits of the activities before you resume your everyday routine.

Specific relaxation

For many Pilates exercises there is a complementary relaxation position that you can adopt following a workout that specifically rests the muscles that you have just been using. For example, after doing curls, which work the abdominal muscles, it is important to rest these muscles by clasping your knees to your chest for a few moments (see page 103). The kneeling rest position (see page 122) gently stretches out the entire spine after doing back extension exercises.

Not only do these complementary positions provide the opportunity for a welcome rest after strenuous exercise, they also lengthen the muscles that have been working, thereby preventing loss of flexibility that can sometimes accompany repeated contraction of a group of muscles. For these reasons, it is important not to skimp on the relaxation elements of your Pilates routine; they are integral to your program and just as important as the main exercises themselves.

General relaxation

When you have completed your exercise program, adopt the neutral pelvis position (see pages 50–51). Rest in this way for a few minutes and consciously allow any sign of tension to ebb away into the floor.

You could also take up the relaxation position shown on page 207. Alternatively, adopt the kneeling rest position (see page 122), focusing all your attention on your breathing as you do so.

Pilates & Sleep

Pilates saw his exercise method as a route to all-round health and well-being. While modern Pilates teachers tend to limit their advice to the exercise aspect of Pilates teaching, there is no doubt that performing exercise regularly has a beneficial impact on sleep quality and, conversely, that your sleep patterns can affect your Pilates performance. A body that is tired through physical exertion will achieve sound sleep more easily than one that has been physically sedentary but mentally tense. Regular sleep of sufficient duration (most of us need about seven hours a night) provides a firm foundation for physical performance, particularly of the controlled type of exercise practiced in Pilates.

PROGRAM PLANNER

This suggested exercise program is designed to provide a balanced seven-day program of foundation exercises—designed to be repeated at least once—to teach and build basic strength and skills. Each session starts with breathing and alignment exercises and includes mobilization exercises, hamstring and quad stretches, and a wind-down. You can adapt the elements if you want to provided you maintain a balance between different types of exercises: flexion/extension, stretches/strengthening.

Day	Group 1	Group 2	Group 3
1	Alignment exercises (page 50) with Breathing exercises (page 62)	Head and neck rolls (page 74) Shoulder mobilization (page 78)	Spine lift (page 86)
2	Alignment exercises (page 50) with Breathing exercises (page 62)	Head and neck rolls (page 74) Shoulder mobilization (page 78)	Knee lifts and drops (page 94)
3	Alignment exercises (page 50) with Breathing exercises (page 62)	Head and neck rolls (page 74) Shoulder mobilization (page 78)	Inner thigh squeeze (page 82)
4	Active standing (page 126) with Breathing exercises (page 62)	Head and neck rolls (page 74) Doming and toe wriggling (page 135)	Pedaling (page 138)
5	Alignment exercises (page 50) with Breathing exercises (page 62)	Head and neck rolls (page 74) Shoulder mobilization (page 78)	Spine lift (page 86)
6	Alignment exercises (page 50) with Breathing exercises (page 62)	Head and neck rolls (page 74) Shoulder mobilization (page 78)	Knee lifts and drops (page 94)
7	Active standing (page 126) with Breathing exercises (page 62)	Head and neck rolls (page 74) Doming and toe wriggling (page 135)	Ankle rotations, pointing and flexing (page 134)

Tips for Practice

If you feel tired or under the weather either skip your practice or do a reduced version that is limited to mobilizations and stretches. You can always return to a foundation version of any exercise if you feel overworked.

If you can't practice every day, don't worry: practice when you can, but remember you will progress more slowly.

Group 4	Group 5	Group 6	Group 7
Abdominal curls (page 102)	Back extension (page 106) and rest position (page 122)	Quad stretches (page 118) Hamstring stretches (page 98)	Chest opening (page 202)
Hip rolls (page 50)	Prone inner thigh squeeze (page 114)	Quad stretches (page 118) Hamstring stretches (page 98)	Full body stretches (page 206)
Abdominal curls (page 102)	Back extension (page 106) and rest position (page 122)	Quad stretches (page 118) Hamstring stretches (page 98)	Roll downs (page 130)
Roll downs (page 130)	Ankle rotations, pointing and flexing (page 134)	Quad stretches (page 118) Hamstring stretches (page 98)	Full body stretches (page 206)
Hip rolls (page 50)	Back extension (page 106) and rest position (page 122)	Quad stretches (page 118) Hamstring stretches (page 98)	Chest opening (page 202)
Abdominal curls (page 102)	Prone leg stretch (page 110)	Quad stretches (page 118) Hamstring stretches (page 98)	Breathing practice in the rest position (page 122)
Knee lifts and drops (page 94)	Prone inner thigh squeeze (page 114)	Quad stretches (page 118) Hamstring stretches (page 98)	Roll downs (page 130)

Your Personal Program

Self-discipline
You will need to engage your mental powers to stick to your planned exercise program.

The exercise program on the previous pages is designed to provide a balanced structure to your practice. Although it is based around a seven-day sequence, you can practice on alternate days if your daily routine does not allow for more frequent sessions. You will still progress, albeit more slowly. Repeat the seven-day sequence at least once before thinking about extending your practice.

Longer sessions

The daily program is designed to be short, because most people don't have time for a long session every day. If you have time and energy you can add extra foundation exercises to your program. But make sure that you practice all the exercises equally and do not overtire yourself—this may ultimately be counterproductive. With longer practice you may build your strength more effectively, but it is still advisable to spend a minimum of 14 days on your foundation program. This gives your body the chance to assimilate the new habits you are teaching it.

Preparing to progress

After 14 days of practice, you may wish to review your progress. Read the self-assessment guidelines on page 140 before deciding to move on. If you feel confident that you are ready to extend your practice, add one of the additional exercises (see the box at right) to your daily practice. When you feel that you have mastered a foundation exercise, you can then substitute its progressed version. It's probably best not to include more than one new exercise in any one session—integrate new exercises into your program gradually.

Additional Exercises

The following progression exercises can be added to your program when you feel ready:

Four-square breathing (page 146)

Turned-out knee raises (page 162)

Arm raises and rotations (page 186)

The Spring (page 190)

Seated side stretches and rotations (page 194)

Side leg lifts (page 198)

Choosing your Progression Exercise

Foundation exercise	Progression
Spine lift (page 86)	Spine lift with overhead stretch (page 151)
Abdominal curls (page 102)	Progressed abdominal curls (page 166) The Hundred (page 170) Diagonal shoulder raise (page 174)
Back extension (page 106)	The Javelin (page 182)
Hip rolls (page 50)	Double knee lift and roll (page 154)
Prone leg stretch (page 110)	Diagonal stretch variations (page 178)
Prone inner thigh squeeze (page 114)	The Javelin (page 182)
Roll downs (page 130)	The Spring (page 190)
Hamstring stretches (page 98)	Seated hamstring stretches (page 158)

FOUNDATION EXERCISES

The exercises in this chapter provide a sound foundation for any newcomer to Pilates. They act as a warm-up as well as a gentle introduction to the strengthening and realignment of the body, which is the ultimate aim of your Pilates journey. Don't expect to master all of these exercises right away. It may take several weeks of practice to perform them all with confidence, and you certainly won't have time to complete more than a small part of them in a single session. Remember to vary your program to include all of the exercises on a regular basis. Every body has its own strengths and weaknesses, so it is normal to find some exercises easier than others. Remember to read the cautions outlined on page 36 before you start.

Mobilizing the Neck

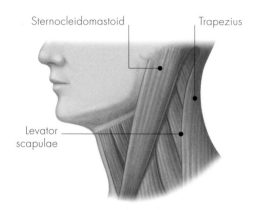

Sternocleidomastoid

Trapezius

Levator scapulae

Principal muscles
The neck is supported and mobilized by muscles that connect the skull, vertebrae, collar bone, and shoulder blades.

Pilates exercise encourages you to create a long neck that is able to support the weight of the head in a completely balanced way. This improves your appearance, reduces strain on the neck muscles and bones (cervical vertebrae), and contributes to the overall alignment of the spine.

The neck muscles

The muscles that are involved in moving the neck are:
- The sternocleidomastoid, which is the prominent muscle that runs from the ear to the front of the base of the neck. This muscle enables you to turn your head and pull it forward.
- The trapezius, which is attached to the top of the spine at one end and to the shoulder blade at the other. This lifts the shoulder.
- The levator scapulae, which is attached to the vertebrae in the neck and to the shoulder blade. This stabilizes the shoulder blade, while the arm moves.

Neck stiffness

Each of the neck muscles easily becomes tense and stiff in people who have stressful, sedentary jobs. Once you are aware of this problem, it is easy to catch yourself bringing your shoulders up toward your ears at times of anxiety or concentration. Neck tension in turn leads to hunching of the shoulders and may be a contributory factor in recurrent headaches and back pain. Mobilizing your neck muscles helps to rid yourself of such tension and the problems it causes. Releasing neck tension can help to improve posture and relieve recurrent aches and pains.

Releasing the neck

In order to start using the neck muscles correctly, you first need to release any tension that they may be holding, because this may restrict or distort your freedom of movement. The exercises shown on the following pages are performed in the supine (lying down) position. This pose allows you gently to stretch and mobilize the neck muscles in a position where they do not need to support the weight of the head. Make sure that you perform these movements slowly and with concentration, as rapid movement of the head and neck carries the risk of muscle strain and possible stress on the joints and cushioning disks between the neck vertebrae.

Take Care

When you try the neck exercises, if you find that moving your neck causes dizziness, faintness, pain, numbness, or tingling in the arms or hands you should stop the exercise immediately and seek medical advice. The movement may have been compressing a nerve or blood vessel in your neck.

HEAD & NECK ROLLS

These simple movements are a relaxing preamble to the more challenging exercises. Perform them in the supine position after you have rested in the neutral pelvis position for a few moments. As with many Pilates exercises, you must not be deceived by the apparent simplicity of the movement required. You need to concentrate and engage your powers of body awareness to be sure that your exercise is having the effect that it should. Make sure that you breathe naturally and easily throughout the exercise.

1 *Lying in the neutral position (see page 51), looking straight ahead, breathe in and out a few times. Focus on relaxing the neck muscles.*

2 *Now roll your head slowly to one side, allowing the weight of the head to govern the movement. Return your head to the center, pause, and then roll to the other side. Repeat the whole sequence five times.*

3 *From the starting position, raise your chin to tilt your head backward.*

4 *Now bring your chin toward your chest so that you feel a gentle stretch in the back of the neck. Slowly repeat steps 3 and 4 five times.*

5 *Return to the starting position and breathe easily for a few moments.*

Shoulder Release

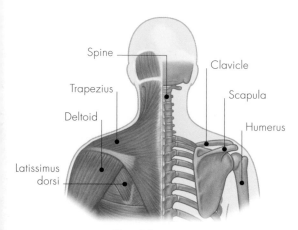

Shoulder structures

The muscles involved in movement of the shoulders are attached to the spine, shoulder blade (scapula), collar bone (clavicle), and/or upper arm bone (humerus).

- Spine
- Clavicle
- Trapezius
- Scapula
- Deltoid
- Humerus
- Latissimus dorsi

Once you have released the neck area, the next step is to start the process of freeing and realigning the shoulders. We have already seen how tension can be focused in both the neck and shoulders. At times of mental and emotional stress the shoulder muscles tighten and over time become shortened, which pulls the upper body out of alignment. Hunched and rounded shoulders limit the expansion of the chest and therefore have a restrictive effect on breathing. Add to this the problems caused by crouching for long periods over a desk that may be the

wrong height, and the strain and long-term distortion caused by carrying heavy loads such as bags of groceries or a heavy briefcase—always in the same hand—and the result is one in which free and balanced movement of the upper body and arms is a virtual impossibility. However, it's possible to get your shoulders back to how they should be.

Benefits of shoulder release

In Pilates it is a key principle that the shoulders should always be relaxed downward. When you hold your shoulders correctly in this way your entire spine, from neck to pelvis, lengthens. The ribcage is also freed up, which allows greater expansion of the lungs and therefore creates more effective breathing. When the shoulders are mobile and stabilized through appropriate exercise, the range of movement of the arms is increased and the risk of strain is reduced.

Visual indicators

The tops of the shoulders can be seen easily if you look into a mirror, so it is relatively straightforward to spot when they are hunching up toward your ears or if one is raised higher than the other. A few shrugs that allow the shoulders to drop down from the ears will often help to release this area.

You are probably less aware, however, of the position of your shoulder blades. When you are tense these tend to ride up the back, which contributes to a round-shouldered appearance. When realigning the shoulders, a prime consideration is to develop a sense of the shoulder blades "sliding down" the back toward your waist. Once you have taught yourself to recognize when this is happening, you should make it your mission to remind yourself to keep your shoulder blades dropped at all times. Try checking every ten minutes or so to see if your shoulder blades are still in a dropped position— you will soon come to recognize how to tell if they start riding up again.

SHOULDER MOBILIZATION

The initial exercise for adjusting the shoulders is a simple, vertical arm stretch and dropping movement, which eases out tension and allows the newly relaxed shoulder to fall back into a more natural position. The exercise then progresses to an overhead stretch. All of this is done in the supine position, which helps to support the rest of the body while you focus on the shoulders. Rest your head on a folded towel or thin pillow if you wish.

1 *Lying in the neutral position with your arms at your sides, visualize your body lengthening without strain, from head to toe. Breathe into the ribs and as you breathe out raise your arms vertically with the palms facing each other. Stretch your arms up as if you were being pulled by your fingertips, but keep your elbows soft.*

2 *Take another in-breath and stretch one arm further to lift the shoulder blade from the floor.*

3 *On the out-breath, allow the shoulder blade to drop back to the floor, keeping the arms raised. Be aware of how your shoulder position has changed. Alternating sides, complete a total of five repetitions on each side.*

4 *Return to the neutral position. Breathe in and engage your centering muscles. On the out-breath, lift one arm overhead, keeping it extended but soft at the elbow.*

5 *Take the arm only as far as you can without arching your upper back—for beginners this is usually to the level of your ears. Keep your ribs and shoulder blades relaxed down toward your waist. Bring the arm back on an in-breath. Note: If your arm can't comfortably touch the floor, place a cushion behind your head to support it at the end of the movement, then allow it to relax into the floor for a few breaths. Alternating sides, complete a total of five repetitions on each side.*

Concentrate on keeping your upper torso stable throughout this movement

Be conscious of your shoulders relaxing downward

Isolating the Inner Thigh

Inner thigh muscles
*These important muscles need to be
both strong and free from stiffness to
allow ease of leg movement.*

Psoas

Quadratus
lumboram

Sartorius

Learning to identify separate groups
of muscles, and mastering how to use
them independently, is an important
aspect of Pilates that is known as
isolation. Most of us use our bodies
without any consciousness of the precise
muscles that we are engaging in the
course of any movement. We operate
on the basis of automatic and habitual
patterns of movement that scarcely
impinge on our thought processes. And it
is often true that the muscles used in our
movements are not those that are the most
efficient for that action, or that we actually

use muscles that are unnecessary and
therefore create needless fatigue.

As you become proficient in Pilates,
your awareness of the actions of your
body will increase and you will learn
how to control your movements to bring
the muscles you want to use into play for
any particular action that you wish to
undertake. As a result, your movements
will become more economical, harmonious,
and graceful. You will also be less prone
to injury because your actions will be less
haphazard. You will be much more in
control of your body and what happens
to it as you move around.

Inner thigh & pelvic floor

Among the muscle groups that many of us
have lost conscious control over—with the
result that they are underused—are those
of the inner thigh and pelvic floor. When
asked to engage them, most of us have
a tendency to tense the entire buttock
area as well, which counters the spine-
lengthening and pelvis-stabilizing benefits
of using just the pelvic floor and inner
thigh. The exercise on pages 82–83
is designed to exercise these often-
neglected muscles specifically.

Because of the difficulty most people experience in working these muscles, the exercise is also valuable for improving focus, concentration, and body awareness.

The exercise is intended to work the lower part of the girdle of strength. When you are starting Pilates it is easy for strenuous physical effort to create tension in the upper back and shoulders as you attempt to bring your whole body into the exercise—it is important that you learn to relax. Throughout this exercise constantly remind yourself that the upper body, shoulders, and neck should be relaxed and check for signs of tension regularly in your jaw, neck, and shoulders (see page 77). The groin and fronts of the thighs are other areas where unwanted tension can build up. Check that these areas are relaxed and are kept "soft" throughout the exercise.

Rolled towel
*Use a firmly rolled towel
for this exercise, if you
don't have a suitable
cushion.*

INNER THIGH SQUEEZE
For this exercise you will need a firm cushion or a rolled towel that you will place between your knees and squeeze. It is important that you start the exercise lying with your pelvis in a neutral position (see pages 48–51), and your shoulder blades relaxed downward, and that you employ a general sense of lengthening down the entire spine. The exercise itself may seem simple at first, but it takes time and practice to perfect the art of working only the muscles that are required. Recheck your technique at each repetition. There should be no tension in your upper body or buttocks.

1 *Lie in the neutral position.
Place a cushion or rolled towel
between your knees.*

2 *Breathe in. On the out-breath
engage the pelvic floor, hollow
your tummy, and squeeze the
cushion between your knees using
only your inner thigh muscles. Aim
to hold this squeeze and control
your out-breath for a count of ten.
Repeat the exercise six times.*

Relaxed
upper body

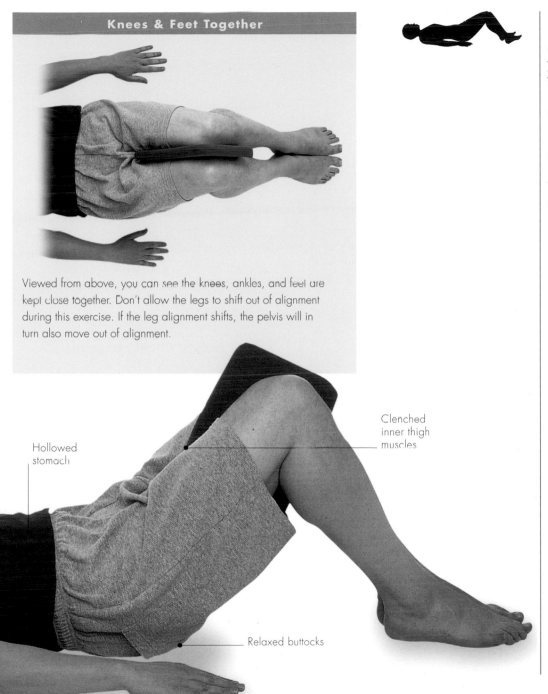

Knees & Feet Together

Viewed from above, you can see the knees, ankles, and feet are kept close together. Don't allow the legs to shift out of alignment during this exercise. If the leg alignment shifts, the pelvis will in turn also move out of alignment.

Clenched inner thigh muscles

Hollowed stomach

Relaxed buttocks

Mobilizing the Lower Back

Quadratus
lumboram

Psoas

Iliacus

Internal abdominal muscles
*Pilates back and abdominal exercises help
to tone and strengthen these muscles.*

B y the time we reach adulthood most of us have lost much of the spinal mobility that we enjoyed as children. A sedentary lifestyle without a range of physical activities usually results in stiff muscles and ligaments in the back. Such stiffness makes us more prone to injury and can lead to chronic back problems. Even those who lead a more physically active life, such as professional athletes, or those who are engaged in some form of physical work on a regular basis, often use their backs in an unbalanced way that creates strain on the structures of the back.

Weak abdominals, weak back

A reduced range of movement in the spine is almost always accompanied by a weakness in the abdominal muscles. Active abdominal muscles control and protect the spine during movement as well as when we are sitting or standing. For this reason, Pilates exercises that are specifically aimed at benefitting the back always involve the abdominal and other centering muscles too.

From pelvic tilt to spine lift

As part of the alignment exercises on pages 50–51, you learned to position your pelvis in relation to the spine to create a neutral position. The spine lift exercise on the following pages builds on this awareness of the alignment of your pelvis and lower back, and helps you to create and control a healthy range of movement in this area. The emphasis here is on locating and using your balanced, neutral position for your pelvis—remember this is different for everyone—and then learning to use your centering muscles to maintain that position while engaging in a range of movements. To achieve this it is important to follow the instructions carefully and to build up the number of repetitions gradually. You need to take time now to ensure that you find the correct position to undertake each of the foundation exercises: one repetition well executed is worth far more than a full number completed incorrectly.

The Power of Visualization

Remember that visualization techniques can be an invaluable aid in the correct practice of Pilates exercises. Everyone needs to develop their own visual vocabulary—an image that helps one person does not necessarily help another (see page 58). In the spine lift exercise on pages 86–87, use whatever image works to guide you.

SPINE LIFT

No matter how long you have been practicing Pilates, there is always a benefit in returning to the basics periodically. Checking and rechecking the alignment of your pelvis and spine is one of these basic exercises and you will encounter it as a recurring element in many of the exercises throughout this book. The spine lift is designed to reinforce correct pelvic positioning and to help you build the strength in your centering muscles needed to maintain that alignment when you are moving as well as when at rest. In this exercise, spinal mobility and lengthening is combined with establishing stability at the center.

1 *Lie down with your knees bent and your feet flat on the floor, hip-width apart. Rest your arms at your sides.*

2 *Breathe in. Then, as you breathe out, tilt your pelvis so that your lower back flattens toward the floor and your pubic bone lifts. Keep your pelvic floor and your abdominals engaged.*

Neck relaxed

Centering muscles engaged

3 As you breathe out, tilt your pelvis in the opposite direction to increase the curve in your lower back. Keep your pelvic floor and your abdominals engaged. Then return to the neutral position. Repeat this process a few times to establish a sense of where your neutral position is.

4 In your neutral position, breathe in. As you breathe out, engage your pelvic floor and hollow your abdomen just enough to curl your tailbone off the floor. Do this by imagining each vertebra in turn, from tailbone to upper back, peeling up from the floor. Try to keep your thigh muscles relaxed and your weight supported equally between your feet throughout.

5 Stop when you have lifted to the point where your thighs and torso are in a straight line and you are resting on your shoulder blades. Hold the position and take an in-breath without relaxing the centering muscles. Then, as you breathe out, reverse the movement, slowly lowering each vertebra in turn onto the floor to return to your starting position. Use your centering muscles to control your body during the entire exercise.

Rotating the Spine

Waist work

Working the external oblique muscles helps to strengthen and tone the waist area.

External oblique

I n the exercise on the previous pages, the focus was on mobilizing the lower spine area in order to create more flexibility and strength by bending the spine forward (flexion) and backward (extension). However, the spine also has the potential to rotate on a horizontal plane (see diagram above). This flexibility of movement allows the upper body to turn to the side while the pelvic area remains stable and front-facing.

Benefits of rotational strength

By controlling and strengthening this rotating movement you can again provide protection against back injuries that commonly occur as a result of excessive twisting of the spine, which can happen when such a movement is unsupported by strong centering muscles. Common activities, such as turning to lift a bag of groceries or to reach a jar in a kitchen cupboard, can easily lead to back strain if you haven't learned to protect your spine by using the whole range of abdominal muscles that are available to you.

Exercises that rotate the spine are particularly important; they release tension in the middle back and stretch out the muscles of the sides and waist area. This part of the back often becomes compressed during long periods of sitting and therefore exercises that mobilize it often provide immediate benefits in terms of relieving minor aches and stiffness. By learning how to rotate your spine you should notice your body becoming less stiff very quickly.

Foundation Exercises **Rotating the Spine**

Multipurpose exercise

Few exercises in Pilates have a single purpose, and rotational work for the spine is no exception. In addition to mobilizing and stretching the back, you will also be developing your external oblique abdominal muscles as they work to control the movement of your pelvis. These muscles are often underused in normal activities. As they become more active and toned, you will be increasing your ability to stabilize your upper torso while moving the area below the waist from side to side independently, in addition to strenghtening the waist area.

Reap the benefits

One of the principal benefits of performing rotational work is that in stretching and strengthening the oblique muscles you promote the lengthening of the waist area. This reduces pressure on the lower spine and over time helps to create a more streamlined outline to your body. It is advisable to approach these exercises with caution if you have an existing back problem.

HIP ROLLS

Do not be overambitious when you first try this exercise. It looks simple, but it is very deceptive. The measure of success is not how far you can drop your knees, but whether you can control the independent movement of your pelvis while maintaining the stability of the upper body. Key points to remember while doing the exercise are: keep your knees and ankles together (visualize them as a single "leg"); keep both shoulders on the floor; and keep your centering muscles engaged throughout the movement.

1 *Lie on the floor in the neutral position. Stretch your arms out to the sides.*

2 Bring your knees and ankles together. Breathe in and engage your centering muscles to hollow your stomach area.

3 As you breathe out, use your abdominal muscles to lift your left hip and tip your knees toward the right. Do not allow your knees and ankles to slide apart. Keep the outer edge of your right foot on the floor and allow your left foot to lift up completely. Keep both shoulders on the floor and stop when you feel your left shoulder beginning to lift.

4 Breathe in and then, on the out-breath, bring your legs back to the center. Control the entire movement with your centering muscles. Repeat the whole process on the other side. Then complete five repetitions on each side.

Isolating the Pelvis & Legs

Vertebrae

Psoas

Piriformis

Inguinal ligament

Hip control
A complex arrangement of muscles and ligaments surround the hip joint and control the movement of the legs.

One of the goals that you are aiming for is to stabilize the pelvis in order to encourage and develop maximum freedom of movement of the hip joints and legs. When most people move their legs when walking, for example, they use a lot of movement from the pelvis rather than exploiting the whole potential range of movement of the hip. This tends to pull the pelvis out of alignment and results in stiffness of the hips, because their full range of movement is underused. When you have learned to stabilize your pelvis and increase your hip mobility, you will find that your movements become more economical and you will

therefore tire less easily. Your actions will also become more graceful as your body will be much better balanced.

In Pilates you will learn that stability is not the same as rigidity, in which there is tension throughout the body. You will develop the ability to create stillness in one area by engaging, but not tensing, the relevant muscles. This allows you to move and relax nearby areas without restriction. There is no short cut to achieving this ability but, if you practice the exercises regularly, paying attention to every detail of the instructions, you will soon learn to isolate and stabilize different areas of your body. You will also recognize the sensation of engaging your all-important centering muscles without any tension.

Freeing the hips

In the exercises on the following pages you will develop your ability to move your legs independently of your pelvis, both laterally and forward and back. The objective is not to move each leg very far although, with practice, as your muscles and ligaments lengthen, you will probably find that the distance you can

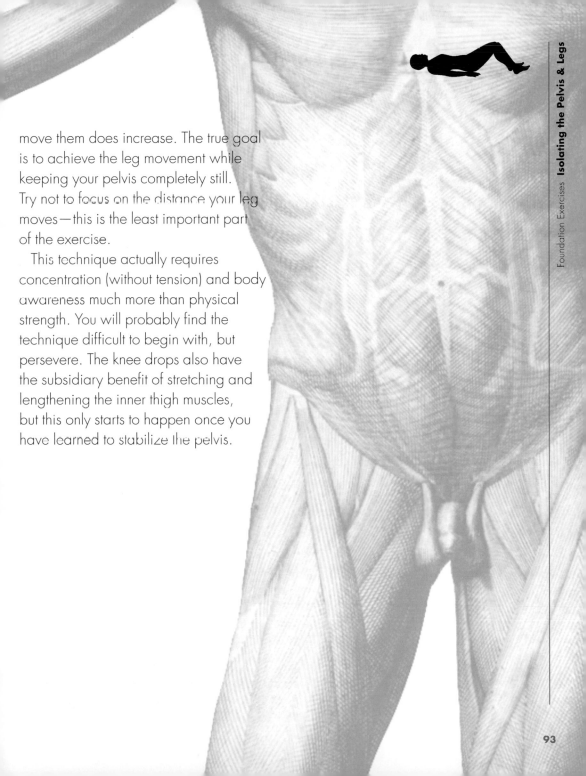

move them do increase. The true goal is to achieve the leg movement while keeping your pelvis completely still. Try not to focus on the distance your leg moves—this is the least important part of the exercise.

This technique actually requires concentration (without tension) and body awareness much more than physical strength. You will probably find the technique difficult to begin with, but persevere. The knee drops also have the subsidiary benefit of stretching and lengthening the inner thigh muscles, but this only starts to happen once you have learned to stabilize the pelvis.

KNEE LIFTS & DROPS

Perform these lifts and drops lying down, in the neutral pelvis position. Spend a few moments renewing your sense of alignment and focusing on the even distribution of your weight over the balance points of the feet. Check that your neck is relaxed and lengthened and that your shoulders are relaxed away from your neck. Be sure to maintain a sense of elongation from neck to tailbone throughout the entire exercise.

1 *Start in the neutral position. Breathe in.*

2 *As you breathe out allow your right knee to drop slowly down toward the floor. Keep your pelvis and left leg stable throughout this movement, using your centering muscles. Avoid pressing down too hard on your left foot.*

3 *Bring your knee slowly back to the center on the in-breath, controlling the movement with your centering muscles. Repeat the whole process on the other side. Complete a total of five repetitions on each side.*

Foot relaxed

Stable pelvis

4 *Return to the neutral position. Breathe in and on the out-breath raise your right leg, slowly peeling your foot off the floor to a height of about 12 inches (30 centimeters) and keeping the knee at a right angle. Focus the movement in your hip joint and keep your pelvis stable throughout. Return your foot to the floor on the next in-breath. Repeat on the other side. Complete a total of five repetitions on each side.*

Freeing the Pelvis

Location of the hamstrings

The three hamstring muscles extend from the pelvis down the back of the thigh.

Biceps femoris

Semitendinosus

Semi-membranosus

Contracted hamstrings

Shortened hamstrings

When the hamstrings remain contracted for long periods they become shorter and stiff.

We have seen how Pilates aims to achieve a balance between strength and stability as well as mobility and freedom of movement. In the exercise on the following pages, you will be learning to free the hamstring muscles.

What are the hamstrings?

This group of three muscles runs from the back of the pelvis to the knee and is responsible for bending the knee. The hamstrings can become shortened and inflexible as a result of sitting. When the knees are bent like this the muscles become lazy—they are relaxed, but unstretched. The result is that when we try to adopt a position in which they should reach their full length, movement is restricted. This is shown by the difficulty that most Western adults experience when they try to sit on the floor with their legs extended. Shortened hamstrings also tend to pull the pelvis out of alignment, distorting the spine and flattening the lumbar curve.

Be patient

If you have never paid any attention to your hamstrings before, don't expect miracles in a few exercise sessions. These muscles will probably need regular and gentle stretching over several weeks or more. If you try to rush this process by forcing a stretch beyond comfortable limits, you will not only fail to improve more quickly, but you may cause muscle damage that could make you stiffer than when you started. The correct technique for any stretching exercise is to create a gentle, continuous pull. This should not cause any pain and the stretching sensation should gradually ease as you breathe into the position.

Beware of Bouncing

One thing you should never do is to "bounce" the body part in question in an effort to take a stretch further. This has the opposite effect from that intended, because the overstressed muscle fibers actually contract to protect themselves from damage. So take your stretching exercises slowly in order to achieve the maximum progress possible.

Scarf
You can use a scarf just as effectively as an exercise band for the stretching exercises.

HAMSTRING STRETCHES
The Pilates hamstring stretch is carried out in the supine position, which supports the body during the exercise and allows maximum relaxation. You will need a long scarf or an exercise band to stretch against. Remember that effective stretching should be a relaxing part of your routine. However, this does not mean that you can perform the exercise in a sloppy way; it requires as much precision as any other Pilates movement. Be sure to give an equal stretch to each leg.

1 *Lie down in the neutral position. Bend your right knee and wrap the exercise band, or scarf, under your foot. Take hold of each end of the band with your arms away from your sides. Imagine a straight line from your elbows, through your wrists, and along the length of the band.*

2 *Breathe in. On the out-breath straighten the leg against the resistance of the band. Lengthen your leg as if stretching your heel toward the ceiling. Take the stretch as far as is comfortable, raising your leg toward the vertical position. Don't lock the knee. Breathe easily through the stretch, keeping your whole body relaxed and your weight evenly supported on your left foot. Repeat on the left side.*

Viewed from Above

From this overhead point of view you can see the elbows are held away from the sides of the body. Also note that throughout the entire stretch the raised foot is directly above the hip. The supporting leg is relaxed and placed in line with the body.

Strengthening the Abdominals

Transversus abdominus

External oblique

Rectus abdominus

The abdominal muscles
These muscles provide support for the entire torso, including the back.

t will be clear by now that strengthening the abdominals is the key to successful body control. Virtually all Pilates exercises involve the centering muscles, which includes the abdominals, to some extent. There are, however, certain exercises that are aimed specifically at building strength in the abdominal area. The abdominal curls on the following pages should become a key element in your Pilates program. With regular practice your strength and control will improve.

The muscles

Traditional sit-up exercises focus on the rectus abdominus muscle, which forms the vertical layer of muscle in the center of the abdomen, most familiar as the "six-pack" muscle. This muscle helps to curl the head and legs in toward the center of the body. Pilates curls also engage the transversus muscles that run horizontally from the center of the abdomen to the spine. The combined action of the muscles has a flattening effect on the abdomen. The abdominal curl also emphasizes the deeper muscles of the abdomen, which provide support and strength to the back.

The abdominal muscles often become ineffective through lack of use. They can also become slack as a result of excessive weight gain or poor posture, both of which stretch and weaken the muscles. In some cases the abdominal muscles seem well developed, but nevertheless fail to provide effective support for the back and abdominal organs. This can be caused by performing abdominal exercises without effectively pulling the navel to the spine. The rectus abdominus then dominates the exercise, bulging outward and preventing the transversus muscles from becoming fully engaged.

Achieving abdominal strength

The abdominal curl demands concentration and attention to detail. Performed correctly it will strengthen and flatten the abdomen. It is very important that you do not attempt to work beyond your strength or you will be unable to maintain the precision of your movements and may strain your back and neck, or start to work the wrong muscles. As long as your stomach is hollowed throughout the curl, your spine will be protected and your rectus and transversus abdominus muscles will be working together correctly. Stop as soon as you are unable to maintain a hollow stomach.

ABDOMINAL CURLS

There are many variations on this exercise so if you attend a Pilates class you may find that your teacher uses a slightly different version than the one shown here. However, there are two elements that all Pilates-style abdominal curls have in common: the emphasis on hollowing the stomach during the entire movement and the need to coordinate the effort with an out-breath. It will help if you visualize the path of the movement of the head as an arc. Remember to work within your own limits.

1 *Lie on your back in the neutral position. Place both hands behind your head. During the curl use your hands to support the weight of your head, not to force or lead the movement with your neck.*

2 *Breathe in. On the out-breath, engage your pelvic floor, hollow your stomach area, and start to curl your chin toward your chest, leading with the top of your head. Visualize each vertebra peeling off the floor in turn. Keep your chin in a neutral position and make sure your neck and throat are relaxed and your shoulders are down. Direct the movement toward the center of your body, with your ribs and the muscles in your upper abdomen pulling down toward your navel and your lower abdominals in toward your waist. Keep your pelvic floor engaged.*

Release

When you have completed your set of abdominal curls, adopt the release position. Take hold of your knees and pull them toward your chest. Breathe steadily, feel your spine lengthening, and allow your abdominal muscles to relax.

3 *When you have curled as far as you can on the out-breath, hold the position and inhale. On the next out-breath slowly uncurl, keeping your stomach hollow and your abdominals in control of the movement. Repeat the whole exercise six times.*

Working on Your Front

Prone position
This is the starting point for most of the exercises carried out on your front.

The next group of exercises involves working face down in the "prone" position (seen below). In this position you become more aware of the air in your lungs expanding the back of the ribcage. You can also focus on the placement of your shoulder blades and accustom yourself to the way they feel when they

are correctly positioned down your back. This is the best position in which to practice back extension exercises. These strengthen the erector spinae muscle that extends down the spine and those that link the backs of the vertebrae.

Body awareness

Before you start exercising in the prone position spend a few moments lying on your front and adjusting your alignment in this position. Here is a checklist of points to look out for:

- Your feet should be parallel with each other, in line with your hips.

Shoulder blades
relaxed down back

Buttocks
relaxed

- Your pelvis should be level.
- Your buttocks and abdomen should be relaxed.
- The bones of your pelvis should sink into the floor.
- Your ribs should be relaxed downward into the floor.
- Your shoulder blades must be relaxed down your back.
- Your arms should be relaxed, either at your sides or bent so that your hands are by your head.
- Your neck should be lengthened and in line with your spine.
- Your forehead can rest on your hands or on a thin cushion.

Breathing awareness

When you are aligned lying on your front, practice your breathing:

- Breathe in, expanding the back of your ribcage.
- Breathe out, drawing your ribs and shoulder blades down toward your waist, engaging your lower abdominal muscles and maintaining the stability of your lower back.

If you find it hard to know if your abdominal muscles are engaged in this position, place your hand under your stomach, inside the hip bone, and you should be able to feel your muscles engage and relax.

Knees aligned with hips

Feet parallel

BACK EXTENSION

The range of movement of the spine is much less flexible when bending backward (during extension) than bending forward (during flexion). Do not expect to move very far when you are performing this exercise. The important point to remember is to keep your lower abdomen engaged and stable on the floor, while achieving a sense of lengthening in the neck and upper back. Do not push on your arms. It may take a few tries to get this exercise right, but you will know you have done so when you feel a stretch from your neck to your middle back.

1 *Lie on your front on the floor with your feet parallel, hip-width apart. Place your bent arms at your sides with your hands palms down. Rest your forehead on a thin layer of padding such as a folded towel.*

Neck lengthened

Shoulder blades relaxed and down

Stable pelvis

Gaze down

One Step Further

Few of us undertake activities that allow us to incorporate back extension movements into our daily lives and consequently the muscles that govern this action are weak in most people. Therefore be prepared to put in a few weeks of practice with this exercise, in order to build your strength gradually without the risk of strain, before graduating to the more demanding progression of the back extension, the Javelin (see page 182).

2 Breathe in. On the out-breath feel your shoulder blades slide down your back. When you feel a stretch up the back of the neck, lengthen the neck further from the body by lifting the head a little. Keep your gaze turned downward. Return to your starting position on the in-breath. Repeat the whole process six times.

Legs extended and relaxed

Lengthening the Legs from a Stable Center

Gluteus minimus

Gluteus maximus

Quadratus femoris

Piriformis

Buttock muscles

The muscles illustrated above are responsible for working the hip joint and are involved in postural alignment.

The prone leg stretch that follows develops stability and strength in the pelvic area and helps to lengthen the spine and legs. It also builds on your ability to work the hips and legs independently of the torso. This is perhaps the most subtle and therefore most difficult aspect of the movement. You will need to engage your full powers of concentration and body awareness to be sure that you are working as intended.

The gluteals

One of the key muscle groups you will be learning to identify and isolate here are the gluteals. These are the buttock muscles, of which the gluteus maximus is the most important. This is the largest of the three gluteal muscles, and it extends from the sacrum and coccyx to the upper part of the femur (thigh bone). The gluteals control the sideway and backward movement of the thigh. They are also important for maintaining the position of the pelvis and therefore play a vital part in your posture and alignment.

Although this is a powerful muscle group, the gluteals are also notoriously "lazy." It requires considerable effort and concentration to make them work effectively. This can be achieved only by isolating the group of muscles from others that normally help initiate the movements in question, including back and abdomen muscles. When you stabilize the pelvis, the gluteals have no choice but to work.

Hip mobility

Leg movement originates in the hip joint (see pages 92–93). Freedom of movement relies as much on the mobility of the joint as on engagement of the muscles around it. One of the benefits of the prone leg stretch is that it helps mobilize the hip joint by stretching the muscles and ligaments that surround it.

Preparation

Before you start the exercise, spend some time adjusting your alignment in the prone position. In particular, pay attention to the position of your shoulder blades; make sure that they are relaxed down your back away from your ears.

Progression

The prone leg stretch is a preparatory exercise for the diagonal stretch on pages 176–79. When you are confident that you have mastered the basic exercise, you will be ready to move on to the more advanced level.

PRONE LEG STRETCH

This exercise may look simple, but it requires careful coordination of stability at the center and freedom of movement of the hips and legs. Practice the breathing in this position, ensuring that when you engage the centering muscles you are keeping your pelvis in neutral and are not lifting the hips off the floor or tightening the lower back. Try to feel your stomach hollowing in this position.

2 *Breathe in. On the out-breath, hollow your abdomen and engage your pelvic floor. Simultaneously, lengthen and raise your left leg about 2–3 inches (5–7.5 centimeters) from the floor. As you are doing this, visualize that the movement is originating from the middle of the buttock.*

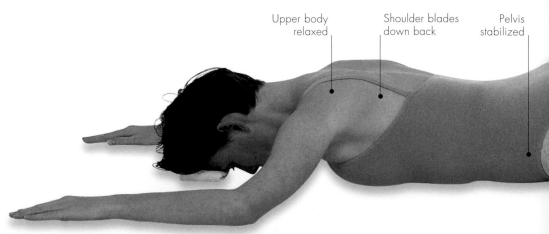

Upper body relaxed

Shoulder blades down back

Pelvis stabilized

1 *Adopt the prone resting position described on page 104. Widen your legs a little and stretch out your arms above your head, keeping your elbows bent. Take a few breaths into your ribs and engage your centering muscles to lift your abdomen toward your spine on each out-breath.*

3 *Lower the leg, still under the control of your gluteals, as you breathe in. Repeat the exercise, lengthening and stretching the right leg. Then, go on to complete four stretches on each side.*

Gluteals engaged

Strengthening the Inner Thigh

Isolating the movement

Effort is concentrated in the buttocks and inner thighs, while the upper part of your body is relaxed.

Continuing work with the muscles of the pelvis, buttocks, and thighs, the next exercise, the prone inner thigh squeeze described on the following pages focuses on isolating the inner thigh and the pelvic floor from the gluteal muscles. These muscles are literally the basis for the girdle of strength—the strong center from which all movement of the body should originate. When toned and active they contribute to stability of the entire torso and, in particular, provide a firm anchor for free movement of the legs from the hips. By working the pelvic floor and inner thigh areas separately from the gluteals, you can work the pelvic floor in more depth.

Small but effective

One of the key features of Pilates exercise is that the effectiveness of the movements is in no way dependent on their size. A very tiny change of position, provided that it is carried out with control and precision will, over time, deliver huge benefits in terms of muscle conditioning and overall body appearance. The prone inner thigh squeeze is an excellent example of this. It engages the muscles at the base of the pelvis against the resistance of a small pillow or rolled towel. Through this almost imperceptible movement you will learn what it feels like to use these muscles and understand how to use them under conscious control. Repeated practice of this exercise teaches the body new habits and enables you to bring these muscles into play—in situations where previously you moved in a way that incurred the risk of strain.

Focus on relaxation

One of the things that many newcomers to Pilates find hard is to relax the areas that are not being worked. Often during exercise we are more used to making an effort using all of our muscles. However, in Pilates the relaxation of key areas during an exercise is as important as the engagement of the muscles in other areas. This is because, in many cases, unwanted tension in a muscle can distort the action of another muscle by subtly altering alignment or resisting the intended movement. In the following exercise it is important to relax the lower legs and feet as well as the upper body and shoulders. As you perform the exercise, constantly check your technique to make sure that tension is not creeping into the areas that should be relaxed.

PRONE INNER THIGH SQUEEZE

In this exercise it is important to lengthen from the waist, up through the spine and down toward the pelvis. At the same time keep your shoulder blades relaxed down your spine. Use a pillow to support your abdomen if you feel your lower back hollowing during the exercise. Maintain engagement of all your centering muscles, but aim to focus the main effort in the inner thigh area. Do not let muscle tension spread to your lower legs or feet.

1 *Lie on the floor in the prone position with your forehead resting on your hands. Relax your shoulders downward. Bring your legs together and place a pillow or rolled towel between your upper thighs.*

Shoulders
relaxed

Shoulder blades
down back

Lengthening
from waist

Progression

Along with the back extension exercise on page 106, the prone inner thigh squeeze forms part of the preparation for the Javelin exercise (see page 182). Make sure you can complete this exercise completely accurately before attempting the more demanding Javelin. This will prevent unnecessary strain and possible injury. Remember also to relax before starting an exercise since this has a dual effect: harmonizing your mind and body makes it easier to focus, and the spine lengthens more effectively when the surrounding muscles are relaxed.

2 *Breathe in. On the out-breath engage your centering muscles and hollow your abdomen to support your lower back. At the same time squeeze the pillow with your inner thigh muscles and then engage your buttock muscles. Keep your feet relaxed and resting on the floor. Relax back to the normal position as you breathe in again. Repeat the whole process ten times.*

Engaged buttocks and pelvic floor

Clenched inner thighs

Freeing the Fronts of the Thighs

Pelvis **Hip joint**

Femur

Quadriceps

Kneeling stretch

Kneeling can be difficult if your quadriceps muscles are shortened. Regular stretching increases your flexibility.

You have already learned to stretch the hamstrings at the back of the thigh (see pages 98–99). However, you also need to stretch the muscles at the front of the thigh. These muscles are known as the quadriceps, or quads. These particular muscles work in opposition to the hamstrings. Contraction of the quadriceps extends the leg, straightens the knee, and lifts up the thigh. Relaxation of these muscles allows the knee to bend fully and permits freedom of movement of the hip joint.

Causes of quad shortening

Both underuse and overtraining can result in stiff and shortened quads. Cycling, in which the quads are under almost constant tension, is an example of a sport that can cause shortening of the quads unless regular counterbalancing stretches are performed. Shortening of the quads may also result from or contribute to postural problems linked to misalignment of the pelvis. The result of shortened quads is reduced flexibility in the knees and stiff movement of the legs.

Choosing your stretch

There are several different techniques for stretching the quadriceps. Choose from those that are shown on the following pages to find the one that you feel most comfortable with or alternatively vary your choice of exercise to avoid monotony in your Pilates program.

All quad stretches rely on maintaining an immobile pelvis to provide a firm base from which to work the muscles. As with other stretches, the quad exercise should provide a gradual lengthening of the muscle fibers. Never "bounce" into the stretch in a misguided attempt to maximize the effect. The result will be further shortening because the muscle tenses to protect itself against further strain. Therefore you should take the stretch only as far as is comfortable for you. As you hold the position, breathe steadily and use your exhalation to boost the degree of relaxation and take the stretch a little further. But don't be overambitious—stop if you feel any pain at all. Take special care if you have a tendency to suffer from knee problems, since most quad stretches involve bending the knee. It is often best to seek expert advice before you embark on such exercises if you know you have a history of problems.

QUAD STRETCHES

Three alternative quad stretches are shown here. Don't do them all during a single exercise session. Instead, choose whichever you feel most comfortable with. If you suffer from knee problems, the standing stretch is most suitable. Hold each stretch for a count of 20, breathing easily and steadily throughout. Try to release tension in your body as you perform the stretch.

Kneeling quad stretch

Kneel with your knees together. Place your hands behind your hips and relax your shoulders. Breathe in and on the out-breath use your centering muscles to tilt your pelvis upward. Feel the stretch in the fronts of the thighs. Repeat five times.

Prone quad stretch

Start in the prone position. Keep your pelvis stable and "rooted" to the floor throughout. Bring one foot back toward your buttocks. Catch the foot with your hand if you can reach or with a scarf if you can't. Pull your heel slowly and steadily toward the center of your buttocks. Feel a gentle stretch in the front of the thigh. Repeat on the other side.

Standing quad stretch

Stand with your feet hip-width apart. Have a chair or other support by your side. Engage your centering muscles and grasp one foot. Keep your pelvis aligned and neutral and your knees together as you bring your heel toward the center of your buttocks. Maintain a sense of lengthening throughout. Repeat on the other side.

Shoulders
relaxed
and down

Hips
level

Chair or
similar support

Knees
together

Lengthening the Spine

Comfort & relaxation
*If your knees are stiff, support yourself
in the rest position with cushions.*

In a well-designed Pilates program the exercises are selected to balance effort and relaxation in each group of muscles. This important principle ensures that muscles that have worked hard do not overshorten as a result of the effort. A counterbalancing stretch during your Pilates session will ensure that the muscles are lengthened as well as toned to provide maximum mobility alongside increased strength.

Many of the prone exercises described on the previous pages involve the extension of the spine. These movements can be strenuous and demanding so the final element of the prone exercises provides a welcome and relaxing counterbalance, incorporating an effective spinal stretch that flexes the spine and releases any muscle tension that may be evident in the muscles that link each of the individual vertebrae.

Relaxation

It is often difficult to be able to relax if you are uncomfortable. If you are feeling pain in any part of your body, this will set up tension throughout the rest of the body, preventing the muscles from relaxing and lengthening. It is therefore important that you do not experience any discomfort when performing muscle-releasing exercises.

For the exercise on pages 122–23 there are several ways you can ease any discomfort you may feel. For example, your knees may be stiff, so try placing cushions under your knees and ankles and/or between your calves and buttocks. Using such support does not in any way diminish the value of the exercise. Experiment to find out which arrangement works best for you, then use it during the exercise. While you are in the relaxation position you can practice your rib breathing, which will increase the stretch to the back. As you breathe in, expanding your lower ribs out to the side, imagine that you are trying to burst out of your T-shirt. Then, on the out-breath, let the ribs release and gently engage the centering muscles.

Completing your relaxation

The way in which you get up from
a relaxation position is sometimes
as important as how you perform it.
After all, there would be little purpose
in spending time releasing tense muscles
if you misuse them as soon as the exercise
session has come to an end.

It is possible to prolong and reinforce
the positive effects of the rest position by
paying particular attention to how you
return to the upright position afterward.
The instructions on the next page include
guidance on how to get up after you
have completed this exercise. There is
also a lying-down variation if you
have knee problems.

REST POSITION

Use this position to stretch out the spine after you have worked your back in the prone position. Although it is intended to be relaxing, the position nevertheless requires the engagement of the centering muscles. This action gently flexes the spine, releasing tension in the muscles and ligaments that link the vertebrae. You should feel a satisfying stretch that lengthens the spine from the lumbar area when doing this exercise. Two versions of it are shown here: the classic unsupported position and an alternative stretch lying on the side. The latter position is best for those who have knee problems.

1 *Kneel on all fours, knees directly under your hips and hands under your shoulders.*

2 *Move your buttocks back toward your heels and sink down so that your forehead is on the floor. Keep your hands in their starting position. Breathe in and feel your spine lengthening. Rest in this position for a few breaths.*

4 *Flex your feet and adopt a squatting position, keeping your centering muscles engaged. Keep your feet parallel, and on an out-breath roll up to a standing position.*

3 *Get up from the rest position slowly. Breathe in and bring your navel to spine. Uncurl gradually, starting from the base of the spine. Visualize your tailbone moving downward. Keep your shoulders down and uncurl your head last.*

Lying-down Variation

If you have knee problems, you can use this alternative rest position after prone work. Lie on your side with your head supported so that your neck is in line with your spine. With your legs together, bend your knees at right angles to your body. Breathe steadily and relax.

Basic Standing Position

The tripod
*Your weight should be evenly distributed
through these three balance points on
the sole of each foot.*

Standing correctly

Correcting your standing posture is
perhaps the most important contribution
Pilates can make to your daily life. Just
because we all spend time standing, it
doesn't mean that we know how to do it
correctly. In fact, most people's standing
posture includes a long list of faults. Pilates
teaches you how to gradually eliminate
them, but because habits are deeply
ingrained, it will take time and effort to
ensure that you always stand correctly.

One of the advantages of standing
posture work is that you can practice
anytime, anywhere. Think about your
posture when you are standing in line in
a store or waiting for a bus and try the
active standing procedure described on
pages 126–27. Nobody else will notice,
but you will feel the benefit as you reduce
the strain on your back and overcome
tiredness. Of course, after regular practice,
eventually others will notice the effects
because you will look taller and younger,
and be more energetic.

Posture principles

When standing you should be aiming
to reproduce in the upright position the
alignment you achieved in the exercise
on page 50. Working from your feet
upward you should have your:
* weight distributed equally over the
  balance points on the soles of your
  feet (see above)
* feet hip-width apart and parallel
* knees soft and facing forward
* pelvis in the neutral position
* centering muscles engaged
* shoulders away from your ears
* shoulder blades relaxed down your back
* chin held in slightly
* head comfortably balanced directly
  over your spine

Still but active

Simply standing is not a rest position, although when you do it correctly it can indeed be relaxing. To hold your body upright you need to actively engage many different muscles. Inappropriate slackness of any of the vital support muscles can lead to excessive strain on another group of muscles. For example, if your abdominal muscles are not properly engaged when you are standing, your back will be forced to take a greater load. You should therefore aim to engage opposing groups of muscles equally, and without excessive effort, to create a sense of balance and lightness throughout your body. In effect, your static body is poised between rest and action.

ACTIVE STANDING

The active standing exercise shown here will help you to achieve balance and alignment. When you practice at home, work in front of a full-length mirror to see how the adjustments you make are affecting your outward appearance. Once you know how it feels to stand in this way, use this position as the starting point for all of the standing exercises that are illustrated in the book and use it to reestablish your sense of equilibrium after doing them, too.

Heel Lifts & Toe Raises

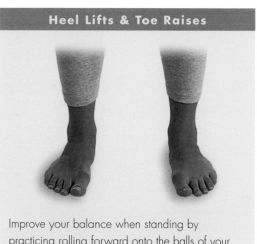

Improve your balance when standing by practicing rolling forward onto the balls of your feet, allowing your heels to lift from the floor, and then rolling back so that your weight concentrates on your heels and your toes lift a little. Engage your centering muscles to stabilize your torso. Use a support for balance, if necessary.

Hips aligned

Knees soft and facing forward

Feet hip-width apart and parallel

Shoulders
dropped away
from ears

Centering
muscles
engaged to
support spine

Pelvic Tilts in Standing Position

To find your neutral position practice a few
pelvic tilts in a standing position.

Tilt the pubic bone
forward to flatten the
lumbar curve.

Tilt the pelvis back
to increase the lumbar
curve. Then return to
a neutral position
between the two
extremes.

Knee bends

*Reinforce your stability and alignment in the
standing position by practicing knee bends.
Breathe in and on the out-breath bend your knees,
keeping them in line with your feet. Bend as far as
you can without lifting your heels. Breathe in and
straighten up. Maintain alignment throughout.*

Spine Awareness

Support & alignment

*Using a wall for support promotes
alignment and precision in this exercise.*

Your spine is not a single unit, but an articulated column that is made up of 33 different bones. To use and develop your back properly, it is important to keep the idea of this segmented structure at the forefront of your mind. Many exercises in Pilates are based on this understanding of the inherent but limited mobility in the back, which is both freed and supported by engagement of the centering muscles in all movements of the torso.

In your exercise program you will be developing your ability to maximize the range of movement in the spine, but also to contain that movement within safe parameters. To do this you need to foster your ability to recognize and control the muscles that are the proper initiators of the action. In particular, you need to develop an appreciation of precisely how working the deep abdominal muscles protects and strengthens your back as it flexes and extends.

The roll down is a classic Pilates exercise, a deceptively simple concept that incorporates the need to carry out a carefully coordinated sequence of actions. It helps to encourage mobility of the spine, and uses the centering muscles to direct and limit the movement. The muscles at the front and back of the body are used in controlled opposition to each other to create the movement while maintaining alignment. The roll down exericse also promotes good balance and an awareness of the distribution of weight through the feet. Your legs also need to be active but should not dominate the exercise; your arms and hands should be relaxed throughout.

Using a wall support

The foundation version of this exercise uses a wall for support and to promote alignment. Practice it in this way until you are able to work with accurate alignment without this guidance. Use whatever imagery helps you to visualize the movement as a gradual "unpeeling" from the wall (or vertical position), vertebra by vertebra from the neck to the base of the spine. The reverse movement, as you slowly straighten up, demands equal physical and mental engagement. The end of the exercise should not be hurried or skimped.

Progression

When you can perform the wall-supported exercise confidently and accurately, try it from a freestanding position. You will need to start from the active standing position on page 126 and use your centering muscles strongly throughout to maintain stability and alignment.

ROLL DOWNS FOUNDATION

Prepare for this exercise by finding a clear section of wall that you can work against. As you place yourself against the wall, check to see if there is any tension in any part of your body, but especially in your back and shoulders. Hold your head and neck aligned over the spine as you begin. Your arms should be allowed to hang without tension by your sides.

2 *Breathe in, relaxing your shoulder blades down your back. Then breathe out, and feel your ribs sliding down toward your waist. At the same time allow your head slowly to drop forward, gradually pulling your spine away from the wall vertebra by vertebra. Allow your arms to follow the movement but keep your knees and pelvis stable.*

1 *Stand by the wall, your feet hip-width away from each other, 12 inches (30 centimeters) away from the wall. Lean your back against the wall and bend your knees a little so that they are in line with your ankles. Check that your pelvis is in its neutral position and your sacrum is in contact with the wall.*

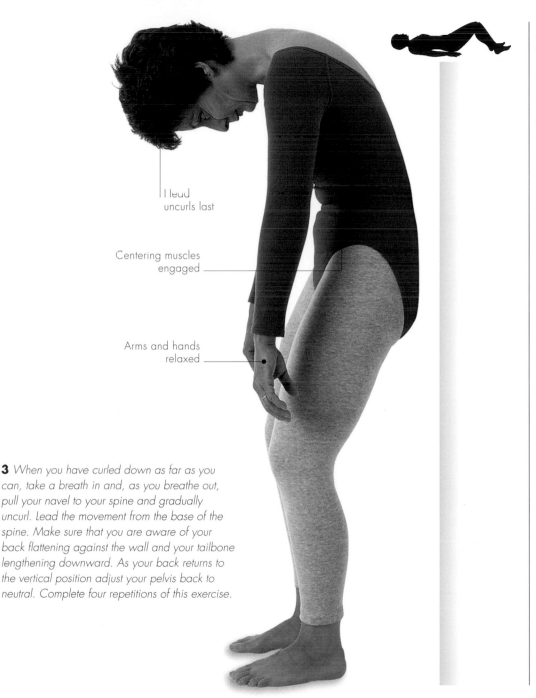

Head
uncurls last

Centering muscles
engaged

Arms and hands
relaxed

3 *When you have curled down as far as you can, take a breath in and, as you breathe out, pull your navel to your spine and gradually uncurl. Lead the movement from the base of the spine. Make sure that you are aware of your back flattening against the wall and your tailbone lengthening downward. As your back returns to the vertical position adjust your pelvis back to neutral. Complete four repetitions of this exercise.*

Groundwork

Phalanges

Metatarsals

Talus

Foot structure
*The numerous tiny bones
in the foot provide maximum
flexibility and strength.*

Your feet are your point of contact with the ground. They provide stability when you are still and are also the launching point for movement. In philosophical terms they can be seen as your link with the earth, connecting you to the source from which all living things originate. However, you don't have to take on board such perspectives to realize that the condition of your feet is fundamental to your overall sense of well-being. Most of us have experienced the huge sense of relief in putting our feet up after a long period of standing or walking. And a good foot massage can produce a degree of relaxation that may seem disproportionate to the area that is being treated. Not surprisingly, therefore, Pilates gives particular consideration to the feet.

Flexibility

The feet and ankles need to be both strong and flexible to support the weight of the body and in order to maintain balance. The complex network of bones and joints in the foot distributes the body's weight over the maximum area of the sole. The inherent springiness provided by the arched structure has effective shock-absorbing capabilities as weight is lifted on and off the feet. However, just as with any other part of the body, the efficiency of the feet can be reduced by years of neglect or abuse. Ill-fitting shoes can also distort and cramp the feet and toes and prevent them from spreading out as they receive the body's weight, which is then distributed over a smaller area. Many of us also spend insufficient time walking barefoot. Lack of this fundamental form of foot exercise can lead to reduced muscle tone in the feet.

₁e Pilates approach

ates foot exercises will help you
rediscover flexibility and mobility in
ɔur feet and ankles. Rotations of the
ɪkles help to restore their full range
movement. Ankle flexibility permits
eater ease of movement through the
ɪgth of the legs and reduces stress on
e back. Repeated flexing and extension
the feet helps maintain muscle tone
ɪd the natural flexibility of the foot
ɪcture. The feet can work harder for
ɪger without aching and they are
ɔle to absorb more of the potentially
ɔmaging jarring forces before they are
ɪnsmitted to the spine. Improved muscle
ɪsponsiveness also makes it easier to
ɔlate the toes, allowing you to keep
em relaxed during exercises when the
ɔt is pointed and to prevent them from
ɪrling back when the foot is flexed.

FOOT & ANKLE EXERCISES
Perform all foot exercises in bare feet. As you rotate your ankles you will need to make a conscious effort to relax. These joints are not used to being idle and tend to tense up as soon as any force is applied. So be patient and give this important mobilization exercise a chance to free your ankles fully. The foot and toe exercises may seem easy until you try them. Most of us are unused to controlling the movement of our toes and the muscles and nerves are often unresponsive to the commands of the brain. The only answer is persistence—you will have to relearn the full potential of your feet gradually.

Ankle rotations
Lie on your back with your knees bent. Lift one leg and support the thigh with your hands. Slowly rotate the ankle six times in each direction. Repeat on the other side.

Toes relaxed

Leg relaxed

Weight on supporting leg and foot

Doming
1 Feet flat on the floor.

Doming |

2 Arch one foot by contracting the muscles on the underside of the foot as if drawing the ball of the foot toward the heel. Keep the toes relaxed and long. Repeat ten times and then do the same with the other foot.

Pointing & flexing
1 Point one foot keeping toes relaxed and long.

2 Then flex the foot back without tensing the toes. Repeat pointing and flexing six times for each foot.

Flexing |

Toe wriggling
Complete your foot and ankle exercises by wriggling your toes to release any tension.

Toe wriggling

Balancing Through the Feet

Weight evenly distributed

Misaligned pelvis

Weight unevenly distributed

Weight distribution
When you stand with your pelvis aligned (left), the weight is distributed evenly over both feet. If one hip is higher, more weight is transmitted down the other leg, unbalancing the whole body (right).

The wider the base over which a load is distributed, the more stable it is. So when we stand with our feet apart we are less likely to topple over than when standing with our feet close together, or only on one foot. It is also harder to balance a moving load than one that is still; constant shifts are needed to keep the center of balance over the main load-bearing area. When we are in action, for example when we are walking, our weight is inevitably shifting; constant adjustments are therefore needed in order to keep our weight evenly balanced over our feet. These little adjustments occur unconsciously most of the time because our bodies have acquired the habit of making such movements. But try altering the load, for instance, by carrying a heavy backpack, and you will become instantly aware of your body having to work to maintain your balance as you walk, stand, and sit. Though your body may unconsciously move to keep you balanced this exercise demonstrates how it can be both stressful on your body and also eventually exhausting.

Minimizing movement
Although your body will have to make adjustments as you move, the Pilates approach to this aspect of body control

is to train the body to keep unnecessary movements to a miminum when you are in motion. This reduces the amount of effort that needs to be expended on adjusting and rebalancing after each step. The result is smoother and more graceful actions that are more economical and therefore less tiring.

In the exercises on the following pages you will be practicing keeping your body, and in particular your pelvis, stable as you shift your weight from one foot to the other. This teaches you to maintain a level pelvis as you walk, which will minimize effort and reduce strain. The second exercise provides additional practice in keeping your balance through changes in your center of gravity. It also promotes flexibility of the foot, which is yet another area of the body where the muscles are sadly underused.

PEDALING

Perform the following exercises barefoot to promote maximum contact between your foot and the floor and to allow the toes to spread and work most effectively. It is easy to do the pedaling exercise without proper control, so make sure that you focus on the detail of the movement and notice and stabilize any movement in your pelvis. Visualize the joints of your hips, knees, ankles, and feet moving freely, while your pelvis and upper body remain in alignment. Remember to practice the second exercise an equal number of times on each side.

1 *Start in a standing position. Breathe in and feel your spine lengthen. Breathe out and engage the centering muscles. Peel one heel off the floor in a smooth movement as the knee moves forward. Lower the heel and repeat on the other side. Repeat five times.*

2 *Now practice alternate heel lifts of each foot in a continuous movement, starting to lift the heel on one side as the heel on the other side is lowered.*

3 *Try to achieve a rhythmic pedaling action, keeping your pelvis aligned and stable throughout.*

1 *Start from an active standing position.*

2 *Shift your weight onto one leg, while sliding the foot of the non-weight-bearing leg behind. Point the toes, keeping them in light contact with the floor.*

3 *Breathe in. On the out-breath, keeping your pelvis and torso stable, bend the weight-bearing knee to exert pressure on the toes of the other foot. Pause for a second and return to your starting position. Repeat five times on each side.*

Self-assessment

Developing confidence
As you progress with Pilates, you will gain an increasing sense of fulfilment from the exercises.

If you have practiced all the exercises for a few weeks, you may find that you are impatient to undertake some new challenges. To help you decide whether or not you are ready to move on, it's a good idea to take a moment to review your progress.

Breathing

By now, you should be finding it much easier to expand and contract your ribcage with each inhalation and exhalation. You should also be finding it more natural to coordinate your breathing with the exercises. If you are still finding any aspect of the breathing difficult you should carry on practicing at foundation level.

Centering muscles

Awareness of the centering muscles and the ability to engage them on an out-breath to hollow the abdomen is a fundamental skill to the Pilates technique. Nearly all of the basic Pilates exercises demand some degree of utilization of these muscles, and by now you should be very familiar with the sensation of the abdomen contracting and supporting your torso. If your control of these core muscles is still unreliable—for example, if your tummy still "domes" when you perform the abdominal curl—then you are not yet ready to advance to the more difficult exercises.

Body awareness

Your body awareness will be increasing and it should now be second nature to adjust your pelvis to neutral before starting any exercise. You should be aware of the position of your shoulders and shoulder blades, too. If you still find it hard to feel when your alignment is incorrect, you may need to spend longer on the foundation exercises.

Pain or discomfort

No Pilates exercise should ever cause you any pain. If this occurs you may have an underlying problem or your technique may be wrong. In any case stop exercising and seek professional advice. Do not progress to the next stage. However, a degree of stiffness is normal, particularly the day after a strenuous Pilates workout— it is generally a sign that you have reached muscles that were previously underused. As you become more accustomed to the exercises this will become less noticeable. Freedom from stiffness following exercises that previously caused it is an indicator that you are ready to progress.

Feeling Good

Whether or not you are ready to progress to a more challenging level, you will almost certainly be feeling the benefits of your Pilates practice. Your body will be feeling longer and lighter, and everyday actions will require less effort. This is your main incentive to continue your practice at whatever level suits you.

PROGRESSION EXERCISES

In this chapter you will be introduced to some more advanced exercises. These require greater control over your breathing and include more complex combinations of movements. Many of them also rely on a basic level of strength in the centering muscles. Integrate these exercises gradually into your regular routine when you feel you are ready to progress further. Remember that your Pilates training is not a race, and there is no glory in attempting exercises that you are not ready for. It is better to devote more time to foundation work than to progress too quickly and run the risk of injury.

Progressing Your Breathing

Breathing into the back

In the all-fours position you can develop your awareness of the expansion of the back of the ribcage during inhalation.

Breathing control should always remain the linchpin of your exercise technique. You will by now have an insight into how the way you breathe affects your whole body, both at rest and during physical effort. You will also be finding it easier to switch to rib breathing as you perform your exercises. Your control of your inhalation and exhalation will have improved considerably and you will also notice that you can expand your ribcage further with the in-breath and contract it more effectively with the out-breath than when you first started.

While Pilates does not improve heart and lung capacity in the same way as aerobic exercise does, you will notice

that you are able to control your breathing more effectively. It will be deeper, so the supply of oxygen to your body will be improved, and the expulsion of waste gases more efficient. This results in more energy and stamina.

Breathing each day

It is easy to build breathing practice into your everyday activities. For example, you can do a few minutes of rib breathing while you are waiting in line or sitting at your desk during a break. As you progress with your Pilates program you will probably find yourself using Pilates breathing techniques naturally to help you use your body more effectively as you exert effort, such as when lifting or turning. You will also find that your movements become more confident and deliberate, which will reduce the risk of injuries caused by uncontrolled actions.

Progression exercises

The four-square breathing exercise on the following pages is designed to improve your awareness of the action of the back of the ribcage during inhalation and exhalation. At the same time you will be using your centering muscles to stabilize the curves of your back. Awareness of the position of the shoulder blades also forms an important element of this exercise.

Insights from Alexander

Many of the breathing techniques taught as part of the Pilates method have much in common with those used in the Alexander Technique. This bodywork system is extremely compatible with Pilates exercises and many people benefit from learning both methods.

FOUR-SQUARE BREATHING

For this exercise you should position yourself on your hands and knees. Take the time to make sure that your limbs are placed in proper alignment before starting the exercise. The overall objective is to keep the lower part of the body stable while maximizing the expansion of the ribcage into the back. This requires you to engage the centering muscles, including those of the pelvic floor, without creating tension in the upper back or shoulders. The neck needs to be held in line with the spine to avoid increasing the lumbar curve of the back.

1 *Kneel on all fours with your hands under your shoulders and your knees under your hips, hip-width apart.*

2 *Allow your back to hollow down.*

3 *Now arch your spine, allowing your head to drop down naturally.*

4 *Return your back to a neutral position between hollowed and arched. This is your starting position.*

No tension in upper body

Neck relaxed and aligned with spine

Pelvis stable

5 *Engage your centering muscles and breathe into your ribs, concentrating on the expansion of the ribcage into your back. Then breathe out, drawing your ribcage downward and inward. Repeat ten times.*

147

Enhanced Spine Control

Spine-lift basics

Before performing any spine lift, check that your starting position is aligned and your spine and pelvis are neutral.

By practicing the spine lift on pages 86–87, you will have been developing your awareness of the segmented structure of the spine. When you first attempted the spine lift you were perhaps hardly conscious of the separate movement of each vertebra. But as you practiced the exercise, increased the mobility of your spine, and listened to your body, you will have begun to appreciate and be sensitive to the capabilities and limitations of your spine. Your ability to stabilize your torso by engaging your centering muscles will also have increased and you will be able to complete the whole exercise with assurance and ease.

The more challenging exercises on the following pages enable you to take control of your spine one stage further but do not attempt them until you are completely confident and at ease with the basic exercise.

The main challenge of the progressed spine-lift exercises consists of using the centering muscles to maintain the stability of the pelvis and not arching the upper back as you raise your arms. The inclusion of movement of the arms in the progressed exercises increases the stretch for the spine—adding a spine lengthening quality—and improves your shoulder mobility. It is important to let the curling motion of the spine be controlled by the centering muscles, leaving the shoulders lengthened and relaxed.

The increased complexity of these exercises demands better coordination of both movement and breathing and will therefore also benefit the overall fluidity of your actions.

Don't be alarmed if you find the exercises difficult to begin with—they are much more advanced than the basic exercises so you will need to work on them gradually (see box). You will find as you practice them you will be able to lift a little higher each time.

Don't forget your feet

Spine lifts are achieved through a combination of the engagement of the abdominal muscles and pressure that is applied through the feet. As you do the exercises you need to support the overall movement by keeping your weight evenly distributed over the tripod of the feet (see pages 124–27 to remind yourself how to do this). Try to keep your legs and feet stable but relaxed throughout the exercises on the following pages.

Advancing Step-by-Step

Approach all new exercises with care. Your previous Pilates practice will have prepared you to some extent for the new movements but they will also involve different challenges. Don't rush into the most advanced version of a staged exercise; take the time to practice the preparatory steps before attempting the full movement. In this way you will avoid strain and maintain steady progress.

PROGRESSED SPINE LIFT

Two exercises are shown here, both of which are extensions of the foundation spine lift on pages 86–87. Do not progress to these exercises until you are able to perform the basic exercise with full control of the movement using the centering muscles. In both exercises use your abdominals, which should be pulled securely from your navel to your spine, to lift and then lower the spine vertebra by vertebra. In the overhead stretch version, the arm lift at the end of the spine lift adds a further spine-lengthening quality to the exercise. The feet-to-wall lift demands more abdominal control than the other forms of spine lift. In both of them, lift only as far as you are able to control.

Spine lift with overhead stretch

Make the basic spine lift more challenging by raising your arms overhead on the in-breath then keeping them there as you roll your spine back onto the floor and into a neutral position.

Spine lift with feet to wall

1 *Lie with your feet, hip-width apart, flat against a wall so that your knees are at right angles. Keep your spine lengthened and avoid curling your tailbone.*

2 *On an out-breath, use your centering muscles to curl your spine a little way from the floor. You will find that you exert pressure through the feet. Uncurl gradually as for a basic spine lift. Repeat four times.*

3 *Now take the lift a little further by exerting stronger pressure through the feet and using your buttock muscles. You can also raise your arms over your head at the end of the movement as on the facing page.*

Centering muscles strongly engaged

Buttock muscles active

Equal pressure through feet

Pelvic Stability

Stable pelvis

With a stable pelvis, movement of the legs is focused in the hip joint, promoting graceful and economic action.

Unstable pelvis

When the pelvis moves as well as your legs, the movement causes stress on the torso and spine.

In Pilates free and effective movement is based on a combination of mobility and stability. Unrestricted movement in a joint is encouraged and developed by stabilizing the area of the body in which it is sited. If the surrounding area moves as well, it "takes over" the movement and the joint does not need to work through its full range. This soon leads to loss of mobility and stiffness. In addition, the inappropriate movement of the part of the body that is supposed to be anchoring the joint creates imbalances and strains elsewhere. The hip joints, which allow for movement of the legs, work through

their full potential only when the pelvis is stabilized by using the centering muscles.

Progressing from the knee lift

The double knee lift and roll described on the following pages is a progression from the knee lift that you learned in the foundation exercises on pages 94–95. Move on to this new exercise when you can perform the foundation exercise easily while maintaining a reliably stable pelvis.

To perform the exercise properly you need to be able to use your centering muscles to control the sideways movement of the pelvis and legs together. The weight of the legs increases the intensity of the exercise. The oblique muscles of the lower abdomen feature strongly in this action. The exercise also relies on the correct use of your breathing to help hollow the abdomen so that the internal abdominal muscles are utilized.

Leading from the hip

The rolling movement in this exercise should originate from the hips, not from the knees. It will help if you visualize your pelvis and both legs as a single unit set in concrete. The spine rotates to allow the pelvis and legs to roll to one side under the control of the centering muscles. The movement continues until the shoulder blade on the other side begins to lift off the floor. When this occurs your centering muscles are no longer in control and you should bring the legs back to the center.

DOUBLE KNEE LIFT & ROLL

In the first part of this exercise you need to focus on effectively engaging the centering muscles as well as on using your out-breath to bring your navel toward your spine, hollowing your stomach. In this position your pelvis is quite stable. Do not start to roll your hips until you are sure that you have achieved this. Remember that the measure of your mastery of this exercise is not how far you can roll to the side, but how far you can roll while maintaining pelvic stability. The distance you can roll will increase with practice, but will only occur as the result of improved muscle control.

1 *Lie down with your knees bent in a neutral position. Spread your arms out to the sides. Keeping your centering muscles engaged, on an out-breath raise one knee so that it is above the hip.*

2 On the next out-breath, raise your other knee and position it alongside the first so that they are lightly touching. Don't allow the ribs and abdominals to "bulge" or "pop up" when you raise the second knee. The knees need to stay together throughout the rest of the movement.

3 Breathe in and on the out-breath roll from the hips toward one side. As you do so turn your head in the opposite direction. Lead the movement with the upper hip and do not let your knees slide apart. When you have rolled as far as you can without the shoulder lifting, return to center on an out-breath. Repeat five times on each side.

Knees and ankles together

Centering muscles control movement at all times

Shoulders in contact with floor

155

Easy Sitting

Hamstrings

You may be surprised to discover that sitting, which is such a normal activity, is a progression exercise. However, bodywork specialists from many different disciplines recognize that people living a Westernized lifestyle, which involves long periods spent sitting in chairs, often have great difficulty in sitting on the floor in a strain-free position.

Small children spend much of their time on the floor—crawling, squatting, playing, and sitting in a variety of positions. Their joints are flexible and their key muscles have not shortened as a result of years of unbalanced activity. Sitting on the floor is natural and beneficial to them, but it is a skill that many of us, as adults, have to relearn.

Extending the legs
To sit comfortably with your legs extended you need well-stretched hamstrings.

Problem areas

The main restriction that stops us from sitting (easily) on the floor with our legs extended comes from shortened hamstrings due to lack of use (see pages 96–99). When these muscles are tight, it is hard to extend the legs and at the same time maintain a straight back when seated. This is because the shortened hamstrings tend to pull the pelvis out of alignment. It also requires very strong centering muscles in order to be able to maintain the spine in an upright position against the pull of shortened hamstrings.

Appropriate exercises

You should already have been stretching
your hamstrings as part of your foundation
routine for at least two weeks. These
gentle stretches continue to be valuable
so you should keep them as part of your
regular program.

The next step is to try sitting on the floor
with your legs extended out in front of
you, feet parallel but slightly apart. Focus
on distributing your weight evenly over
your sitting bones (you should be able
to feel these bones under your buttocks
when you are sitting down). Engage your
centering muscles to lift your back into
alignment. Unless your hamstrings are
very flexible, you will probably find that
it is difficult to keep your legs straight out
in front of you in this position. In this case
you may find it beneficial to use a firm
cushion to raise your buttocks and another
under your knees for support when you
first start to practice the exercises illustrated
on the following pages. It may also be
helpful to position yourself with your back
flat against a wall for added support.

SEATED HAMSTRING STRETCHES

The first part of these exercises involves a seated stretch. It is harder work than it looks and needs to be done with careful attention to your technique to ensure that you achieve the necessary stretch. Spend at least a week practicing this stretch before moving on to the combined hamstring and back stretch. These extension exercises encourage spinal mobility and back lengthening. Again, it is the precision with which you perform the exercise, rather than the degree of movement you achieve, that will produce positive results.

Seated stretch

1 *Sit on your sitting bones with your legs extended in front, knees vertical, and your feet parallel and a short distance apart. If necessary support yourself with cushions as described on page 157. Breathe into your ribs and on the out-breath engage your centering muscles to lengthen up from your hips through your torso. Keep your thigh muscles soft. Repeat this five times.*

2 *Repeat step 1 but on the out-breath also flex your feet and slide your heels away from you. Keep your toes relaxed and feel the hamstrings stretch. Relax on the in-breath. Repeat five times.*

Combined hamstring & back stretch

*Sitting as for the seated stretch, breathe into the ribs
and on the out-breath allow the weight of the head
to round the body forward, visualizing bringing your
nose toward your navel. Allow your back to round
but use your centering muscles to maintain a sense
of lengthening. Allow your arms to come forward
with the movement. Keep your shoulders down and
your thighs soft. Roll forward as far as is comfortable
without collapsing at the center.*

Hip Rotation

Centering muscles engaged

Stabilizing the center

Keeping your abdominal muscles engaged in order to stabilize your pelvis is a key aspect of this exercise.

Several exercises in this book focus on the importance of developing pelvic stability alongside the ability to move the legs independently of the pelvis. This will allow you to engage the correct muscles for the job, rather than overworking unnecessary ones. Each exercise furthers your control of this through different types of movement. While having a similar underlying purpose, the varied actions that are incorporated into each of these exercises mobilize, stretch, and engage different groups of muscles.

The area worked

The exercises on the following pages work the deep muscles of the buttocks. Strengthening these muscles provides much more effective and stress-free movement of the hips and legs. In the long term this may reduce wear and tear on the hip joints, which will thereby help to lower the risk of osteoarthritis in later life. Combined with this strengthening action, the hip rotations gently stretch the ligaments that surround and support the joint. This gradually increases the range of movement of the hip joint and therefore also of the leg.

Feeling the stretch

Hip rotations provide a challenge for the centering muscles, because maintaining immobility of the pelvis is of paramount importance. The pelvis needs to be anchored firmly in the neutral position throughout the exercise. In addition, you are also likely to become aware of the work that is undertaken by the deep buttock muscles surrounding the hip. This may be felt at the time as a dull ache around the joint, and on the first occasion you try this exercise may cause stiffness the following day. When you feel this sensation you know that you have reached some of the forgotten muscles that the Pilates method identifies as being crucial to effective body use.

Isolating the movement

The ability to engage specific muscles to produce a certain movement while relaxing others nearby is a fundamental Pilates skill. In this exercise it is important to remember to keep your toes softly pointed, but not tense. If the toes are "locked," muscle tension is likely to spread up your leg, restricting and distorting the desired movement.

Turning out

Pilates exercise emphasizes movements that promote outward-turning of the legs from the hip joints. This is because most of us tend to turn in too much—for example, when crossing our legs in a sitting position.

TURNED-OUT KNEE RAISES

This exercise is performed lying on your back. Because of the importance of maintaining a neutral pelvis throughout the movement, it may be advisable to perform a few pelvic tilts, as described on pages 50–51, to establish your neutral position before you start. Your arms remain relaxed throughout the exercise, but you may find it helpful to rest your hands on your lower abdomen to enhance your sense of the stability of the pelvic area.

1 *Lie comfortably in the neutral position.*

2 *Breathe out and, with centering muscles engaged, raise one knee. Softly point the toes. Breathe in.*

Softly
pointed toes

Stable pelvis

Rotation
from hip

3 *Breathe out as you rotate the raised leg within the hip joint, bringing the foot toward the other knee. On an out-breath, return to center and repeat five times. Do the same number of repetitions on the other side.*

Further Abdominal Development

Curl with lifted arms
Bringing your arms back from over your head during the abdominal curl is one way of increasing the challenge.

Curl with arms & legs lifted
Increase the demands on your strength further by lifting both arms and legs during the curl.

Abdominal strength is a core Pilates goal. And one of the key groups of exercises that you need to master in order to achieve that goal is the abdominal curl. In the foundation exercises you will have learned the basic abdominal curl with both hands supporting your head. Do not attempt the exercises on the following pages if you are still finding the foundation version hard: for example, if you have difficulty in supporting the movement with your abdominals. Most people need several weeks' practice before they are ready to progress.

Increasing the challenge

There are a number of ways in which you can increase the challenge of the abdominal curl. The first is to lengthen the area that is lifted during the exercise. It requires more effort to lift the shoulders from the floor when the arms are extended than when they are held next to the head. The first exercise on page 166, progressed abdominal curls, incorporates an overhead arm stretch with the abdominal curl. This requires careful coordination with your breathing, but once mastered produces a graceful and satisfying movement.

You can also increase the abdominal workload by lifting your legs. In this position, the feet no longer provide a point of leverage for the movement, so the effort is concentrated in the centering muscles. The second progression exercise, which includes a knee lift, requires concentration and body awareness to be both effective and safe. The movement must be controlled through your abdominals and not forced by straining the neck forward or arching the spine. If you find this exercise too hard, work on the easier abdominal curls for a bit longer.

The final exercise, the combined curl, is a composite of both movements. It provides a really effective challenge for the abdominals.

Don't Forget to Release

Whichever version of the abdominal curl you choose, always end your practice with the release position described on page 103.

PROGRESSED ABDOMINAL CURLS

Before you start these progressed versions of the abdominal curl, check that your pelvis is securely in the neutral position. You will need to maintain this position for the first exercise. In the second and third exercises, the lumbar curve inevitably flattens against the floor. However, you need to maintain a sense of the base of your spine lengthening away from the body. Whichever version you are doing, try to retain a sense of the spine stretching as well as curling. Use your engaged centering muscles to prevent yourself from collapsing in the middle. Remember to stop if your abdomen starts to bulge or the muscles begin to quiver. This means the exercise is too demanding for you and is a sign that you need to lift less far or revert to an easier version.

Abdominal curl with lifted arms

1 *Lie in the neutral position with your arms over your head.*

2 *As you perform the curl in the usual way, lift your arms in an arc so that they are just above the floor as you finish your out-breath at the end of the movement.*

Head raised

166

Abdominal curl with raised legs

1 *Lie with your arms at your sides and your legs raised with your knees above your hips.*

2 *Perform the abdominal curl in the usual way, but you will find that you need to work the centering muscles harder in this position.*

Arms lifted from overhead

Legs raised

Centering muscles control movement

Combined arm & leg lift

When you have worked on the previous two versions of progressed abdominal curls, try combining the two elements in one exercise.

167

Understanding the Hundred

A classic Pilates exercise

The Hundred combines strength, control, and coordination in a single exercise.

Perhaps the best known of all the Pilates exercises, the Hundred finds a place in almost every Pilates-based program. In its original form, as devised by Joseph Pilates, it comprises a demanding sequence of movements that challenges your breath control, your abdominal strength, and your overall sense of coordination and body awareness.

Practice & progress

It takes months of practice to be able to perform the movement in its unmodified form without strain. However, don't be discouraged—you can make a start by practicing some of the modified versions that will gradually build your strength and coordination until you reach the point where it is possible for you to complete the full exercise.

The essence of the Hundred

This exercise relies on the strength of the centering muscles being able to support the weight of the upper body and legs while maintaining the neutral alignment of the spine. Pilates himself performed this exercise with the legs extended and horizontal. But only the most highly trained Pilates practitioners are able to prevent their spine from arching in this position and it certainly should not be attempted by beginners. The higher you hold your legs the less the demands are on your abdominal strength. Therefore, as a beginner, you will need to start with your knees bent. Even when you are more experienced and are able to work with straightened legs, don't let them drop lower than about 45 degrees to the floor.

The name of this exercise derives from the number of repetitions that Pilates recommended. Again this is a final goal to aim for. But, as with all goals, you can't expect to achieve it right away. Aim to build up from 20 to 30 repetitions, which you can perform in groups with a short rest between. Always aim to build on what you have done before then practice until you achieve the whole Hundred.

Breath control

Breath control is not an optional extra, but an integral part of the exercise. Do not increase the number of repetitions beyond the number for which you can control your breathing. With rhythmic, coordinated breathing, the Hundred adds an aerobic element to your Pilates practice and becomes a welcome energizing addition to your program.

PRACTICING THE HUNDRED

On this page several leg positions are shown for the Hundred, from the recommended starter version, to some variations that allow more intense work. The breathing and arm movements remain the same whichever leg position you choose. Keep reminding yourself that total control of your body alignment is the aim. This can only be achieved with practice over time. After completing the exercise adopt the release position (see page 103).

Beginner's position

From the neutral position, on an out-breath, engage the centering muscles and lift your shoulders as for an abdominal curl (see pages 102–103) with your arms stretched forward a little way off the floor. Breathe in for a count of five, moving your arms up and down slightly as you do so. Breathe out for a count of five, moving your arms as for the in-breath. Newcomers to this exercise should aim to complete four to six repeats of this exercise without a break, building up to ten repeats (100 movements of your arms).

Lengthened neck

Flattened back

Intermediate position

The exercise is the same as the beginner's version, but the legs are raised with the knees above the hips, bent at right angles.

Legs extended

Arms extended

Advanced position

The challenge of the exercise is increased by extending your legs. Be sure your abdominal muscles are strong enough to allow you to perform the exercise without arching your back before adopting this position.

Working the Obliques

External obliques

Internal obliques

Oblique layers

The oblique abdominals form the outer two layers of abdominal muscles overlying the transverse muscle layer.

The oblique muscles of the abdomen run diagonally around each side to the mid-line of the abdomen. They are involved in all twisting movements of the torso and are also important for stability of the spine, abdomen, and pelvic area. Well-toned obliques contribute to the development of a slim waist and healthy posture.

Abdominals

You need a basic level of abdominal strength to be able to perform the diagonal shoulder raise that is illustrated on the following pages. Don't progress to working the obliques in this way until you have been practicing the abdominal curls on pages 102–103 for at least two weeks. The combination of lifting and twisting involved in these exercises can easily cause strain if you have not yet acquired sufficient abdominal strength to control and direct the movement safely.

Tips for working the obliques

In the diagonal shoulder-raise exercise (see pages 174–75) the obliques are used to help raise and turn the torso as you lift one shoulder up and, at the same time, twist toward the opposite hip. The challenge here is not how far you can lift, but how effectively you can perform the movement while keeping your belly hollowed and your pelvis stable. Keep in mind the following guidelines:

- Initiate the movement from your center, not your neck.
- Aim your armpit, not your elbow, toward the opposite hip.
- Don't pull the back of your head forward with your hands.
- Keep your elbows wide and your chest open throughout the movement.
- Keep your knees and feet hip-width apart and parallel. If your knees tend

to drift apart during the exercise, grip a pillow or a rolled-up towel between them the next time you try it.

Preparation

Develop your sense of this movement by practicing rolling to each side with your hands behind your head and the lower elbow resting on the floor.

Sports twists

Increasing the strength of your obliques and enhancing the way you use them in conjunction with the rest of your abdominal muscles can improve your overall sports performance and can help to prevent strain and injury. Sports activities that particularly engage the obliques include golf, tennis, and squash, all of which involve twisting movements of the torso.

DIAGONAL SHOULDER RAISE

The diagonal shoulder raise is an exercise that is seen in different forms in many exercise programs. The key to doing the exercise the Pilates way is to focus on hollowing the belly throughout the lift. If your stomach begins to dome during the exercise it is a sign that you have moved beyond the point where you can control the movement. When this happens you are no longer engaging the muscles correctly and there is no value in lifting any further. You should breathe in and relax down before starting your next repetition.

1 *Lie in the neutral position and place your hands behind your head. Breathe in.*

Head lightly supported by hands

Elbows held wide

Front View

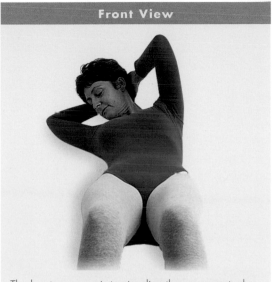

The key to success is to visualize the movement when bringing your armpit toward the opposite knee. Keep your elbows wide to avoid pulling on your neck.

2 *On the out-breath, engage your centering muscles and lift one shoulder off the floor, using your abdominal muscles to initiate and control the effort. Keep your neck relaxed. Do not use your hands to pull your head and neck forward.*

Feet flat on ground

Toward the Diagonal Stretch

Feeling the stretch
*This exercise creates a satisfying stretch up
and down the spine from the waist.*

The diagonal stretch is a progression from the prone leg stretch that is shown on pages 110–11. The movements involved seem minimal, yet again, but as soon as you try them you will appreciate that they are much harder than you ever imagined.

The diagonal stretch strengthens the entire torso. It incorporates work on the shoulder area, stabilizing the structures that support the shoulder joint, which is known as the shoulder girdle. By anchoring this area, the diagonal stretch helps to free the shoulder joint to allow full movement of the arms. The muscles along the entire length of the spine are then engaged. This back extension work avoids the risk of strain because it is fully supported by the abdominal muscles, which are also engaged throughout the exercise. In the lower part of the torso, stability of the pelvis allows the hip joint to be safely stretched as you extend each leg in turn.

Building up gradually

You are ready to progress to this exercise when you feel confident that you can perform the prone leg stretch with ease. That basic exercise will have taught you how to hollow your abdomen while in the prone position and extend each leg in turn while you are doing so.

The next stage is to learn to extend your arms in the prone position, keeping the same hollowing of the abdomen. Be aware of the centering muscles and be vigilant about the position of your shoulders and shoulder blades, which must still be drawn away from the neck. Although you will be extending the arms, they should remain free from tension at all times. The lengthening effect comes from extending the shoulders, not from straightening the arm by muscle action.

When you have mastered arm extension work, try combining the leg and arm extensions in the full diagonal stretch. Here are some key body awareness pointers for this exercise:

- Be aware of your body lengthening from toe to fingertip.
- Feel the stretch originating from the waist and extending up the spine and down through the sacrum.
- Keep your forehead resting on the floor so your neck is relaxed.

177

DIAGONAL STRETCH VARIATIONS

The diagonal stretch is one of the most demanding but also most satisfying exercises. Performed sloppily it will deliver no benefits, but carried out with energy and concentration, you will feel your spine lengthening and strengthening with each repetition. Do not rush to complete the full exercise. Practice the various elements individually to prepare your body for the greater challenge of the combined arm and leg extension.

1 *Lie in the prone position, with your forehead on the floor and your arms extended above your head, and complete a few repetitions of the prone leg stretch on each side (see page 110).*

Shoulder
blades
down back

Waist
lengthened

2 *Lift one arm a little off the floor. Visualize this small movement originating in the shoulder blades, while the rest of the torso is stabilized by your centering muscles. Repeat four times on each side.*

3 *On an out-breath, lift one arm and the opposite leg at the same time. Feel the sensation of lengthing diagonally from fingertip to toe as you stretch away from your waist in each direction. Repeat four times on each side.*

Leg lifted
and extended

179

The Javelin

A straight stretch

*In this exercise you aim to lengthen
your entire body by stretching forward
through the spine.*

In this exercise, sometimes known as the
Arrow, you will be combining the control
learned in the prone inner thigh squeeze
(see page 114) and the back extension
(see page 106). You will need a pillow or
rolled towel to place between your thighs
and an extra pillow to support your
abdomen if necessary. You will also need
a layer of padding for your forehead.

Visualizing the shape

As its names suggest, this is a lengthening
exercise. As you do this exercise, it is
helpful to keep in the forefront of your
mind an image of your body acquiring the
narrow, streamlined shape of a javelin,
spear, or arrow. Often such visualizations
are more effective in directing your body
to adopt the required position than a
series of dry instructions can be.

It is not only the shape of the body that
can be helped by visualization. You can
also direct the way that you use your
muscles by creating a mental image of
the direction of the movement you want
to achieve.

Even in a relatively static exercise such
as this, you will be initiating the movement
of energy in a certain direction. In this
case, the head should be visualized as
moving forward, but your main energy
should be directed through your body
from the neck, along the spine and arms,
down toward the toes. You should also
continue to focus your attention on your
breathing in order to ensure that it remains
slow and deep throughout the exercise.

Isolating the effort

A key Pilates skill in this exercise is
isolation. The muscles of the abdomen,
pelvic floor, back, and buttocks are all
fully engaged to extend and stabilize
the torso. Your limbs and extremities,

however, should remain relaxed. Your hands, feet, and calves should be extended, but free from tension. At each repetition of the exercise, you will need to use your growing body awareness skills to check that your toes and fingers are still "soft" and relaxed. This is important because inappropriate contraction of the muscles in the limbs will act in opposition to the work of the muscles of the torso.

A "lengthened" body

Many exercises in the Pilates system are intended to lengthen the spine. Such exercises activate the muscles of the torso that support the spine, mobilizing and decompressing stiff joints. The result is freer movement and a more upright posture that gives the impression of increased height.

PRACTICING THE JAVELIN

Start this exercise in the prone position. Take the time to adjust your alignment as described on page 104. It is important to do this at the start because the exercise will reinforce any errors in your alignment if you don't. Then perform a few repetitions of the prone inner thigh squeeze (page 114) and the back extension (page 106). This will help you to identify and isolate the key muscles you will be using for this exercise. You are not ready for the javelin if you are still having difficulty with either of the preparation exercises and should spend some time ensuring you are happy with them before moving on to the next level.

Neck
lengthened

Shoulder blades
down back

Waist
lengthened

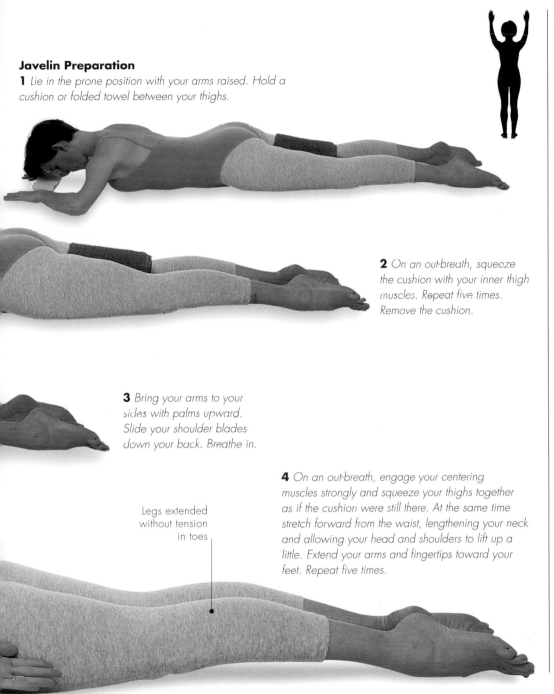

Javelin Preparation

1 *Lie in the prone position with your arms raised. Hold a cushion or folded towel between your thighs.*

2 *On an out-breath, squeeze the cushion with your inner thigh muscles. Repeat five times. Remove the cushion.*

3 *Bring your arms to your sides with palms upward. Slide your shoulder blades down your back. Breathe in.*

4 *On an out-breath, engage your centering muscles strongly and squeeze your thighs together as if the cushion were still there. At the same time stretch forward from the waist, lengthening your neck and allowing your head and shoulders to lift up a little. Extend your arms and fingertips toward your feet. Repeat five times.*

Legs extended without tension in toes

Working the Arms While Standing

Shoulder & chest muscles
Arm exercises involve all the muscles of the shoulders, chest, and upper arms.

Muscles of the upper back
The trapezius muscle works with the shoulder muscles and latissimus dorsi to stabilize the shoulder blades.

Arm exercises may initially look easy and relaxing, however, the reality is that you need to have already achieved a good level of stability of the torso before you can undertake them effectively.

The origins of arm movement

Movement of the upper arm originates in the shoulder joint. This is a highly mobile ball-and-socket joint that, when functioning freely, allows the arm to rotate through 360 degrees. Nowadays, we hardly ever use the shoulder joint to its full potential. All too often we create arm motion by moving the upper body instead of the shoulder joint. This leads to stiffening of the shoulder joint through lack of use, which in turn creates a vicious circle of inappropriate movements that unbalance the body and fail to utilize the full range of its muscles.

Recreating full mobility

Movement of the arm should be initiated and controlled through the muscles of the upper arm, shoulder, and chest. These become active during arm movements when the shoulder blades are stabilized. The exercises on the following pages are designed to help you drop your shoulder blades and stabilize them in this position. Then you will learn to free the shoulder joint and use this newfound mobility to rotate the arm using the correct muscles. This creates active, toned muscles around the shoulders, chest, and upper arms. These exercises also help to counter tension in the upper trapezius muscle.

Posture Reminder

Arm exercises provide a valuable opportunity to recheck and improve your standing posture. They must be carried out from a stable and aligned position, in which the centering muscles are supporting the back and abdomen. Before you start this part of your program, stand in front of a mirror and carefully recheck your standing posture according to the guidelines on pages 124–25.

ARM RAISES & ROTATIONS
Perform the exercises on this page while focusing on immobilizing your torso and dropping your shoulders. It is best to work in front of a mirror so that you can constantly check for signs of hunching of the shoulders, which is the most common mistake. Eventually, however, your body awareness will increase to the point where you can tell immediately if your shoulders are raised because it will feel wrong. Between each exercise in this series, drop your arms down to your sides and shake out your shoulders to release any tension. Then carefully reestablish your starting position.

1 *Adopt the active standing position (see pages 126–27).*

2 *As you breathe out engage your centering muscles and lengthen one arm up to shoulder height with hand and fingers level with the arm. Keep your shoulders down. Bring the arm down on the in-breath and repeat using the other arm. Do six repetitions on both sides.*

3 Using the same technique as in step 2, extend both arms simultaneously. Complete six repetitions, bringing your arms to your sides between each one.

4 On an out-breath, extend both arms out to the sides with flexed wrists. Take an in-breath, then on the out-breath, make three small circles with your arms without locking the elbows. Take an in-breath and then on the out-breath make three small circles in the opposite direction.

5 On an out-breath, extend both arms out to the sides and at the same time come up onto your toes. Use your centering muscles to keep your torso stable. On the in-breath, lower your arms and return to active standing. Repeat six times.

187

Balance & Strength

Center of gravity
For the Spring you need to adopt a semicrouching position in which your weight is distributed evenly around a vertical line through your ankles, hips, and shoulders.

Whether or not it was one of your primary goals when commencing your Pilates program, one of the benefits of this form of exercise that you will undoubtedly be noticing is the improvement in your overall balance and physical coordination. You will find that you are using your body more economically and with greater

sensitivity. In the next series of exercises, based on the Spring, you will be developing your appreciation of your center of gravity and how to use this understanding to provide added stability in your everyday activities.

Stillness in movement

The Spring has its origins in both the yoga tradition and the work of Frederick Alexander, founder of the Alexander Technique. In this position the body's weight is distributed evenly over the hips, knees, and ankles, while the body leans forward and the knees are bent. The position resembles the midway point in the movement between sitting and standing.

The maintenance of this posture requires flexibility of the hips and strength in the torso and legs, as well as a sensitivity to shifts in your center of gravity. Firm engagement of the centering muscles is required to maintain the alignment of the spine, but the tops of the shoulders should be relaxed downward at all times to give an overall sense of ease and energy. The posture is still but many muscles are actively engaged in readiness to "spring" forward when in this position.

The Spring

One of the benefits of practicing this position is that you can begin to use it in your everyday activities. It has already been noted that the Spring is a transition point between sitting and standing. You will be moving in a healthier way if you consciously aim for this position each time you sit down or get up from sitting. Engage your centering muscles, lead with your head, and actively use your leg muscles to control the overall movement. Activities such as lifting and bending will also become less stressful as a result of your familiarity with this exercise.

Once you have established how to maintain the Spring position without strain, you can also use the further exercises on the following pages to tone the muscles in the backs of the arms and between the shoulder blades.

THE SPRING

You may need to prepare yourself for the Spring by practicing a preparatory exercise that uses a wall for support. This will help you achieve the correct angle in which to balance your weight over your legs. Once you have a sense of how the position should feel, try it without the wall to support you and then move on to the triceps squeeze and shoulder rotations.

1 *Stand with your feet hip-width apart, about 6 inches (15 centimeters) away from a wall. Bend your knees slightly and rest your back against the wall.*

2 *Now start to hinge forward from the hips, keeping your back flat and your neck long. Allow your arms to follow the movement.*

3 As you hinge forward your buttocks will come away from the wall and you will be resting in the balanced Spring position. Use your centering muscles to keep your back aligned and torso stable.

4 On an out-breath bring your palms together behind your back. Repeat the movement five times.

Head and neck in line with spine

Arms relaxed

Centering muscles engaged

Weight balanced through feet

5 Finish the exercise by rotating your shoulders in each direction and shaking out your arms and hands.

191

Sitting without Stress

Mistakes
The two sitting positions shown here—slumped and overarched—are equally stressful for the spine.

Most of us spend a great deal of the day sitting down at a desk or in front of a computer workstation, so it is vitally important to adopt a correct sitting posture. Sitting is one of the most stressful positions for the spine. This stress can be reduced if attention is paid to spinal alignment.

From sitting to stretching

The stretching exercises discussed on the following pages are all carried out in a seated position. They are therefore ideal for releasing back tension while you are at work, and can be performed at regular intervals throughout the day. But before you can start on these, you will need to check and adjust the way that you normally sit. The objective is to ensure that the weight of the head is evenly transmitted down the spine and through the pelvis. If you slump so that your back is rounded or, alternatively, over-straighten so that the lumbar curve is excessive, the weight will create stress in parts of the spine. In the long term, back trouble is the likely consequence of sitting in such positions. By supporting your spine in the neutral position, with the muscles of the torso actively engaged, you can minimize the potential for strain or for compression of the disks that provide cushioning between the vertebrae.

A balanced sitting posture

The following is a checklist in order to ensure you are sitting correctly.
- Choose an upright chair that has a firm seat.
- Your feet should be able to rest comfortably flat on the floor with your knees at right angles.
- Sit down with your buttocks near the edge of the chair—your knees should be hip-width apart and your ankles

should be placed directly under your knees.

- Feel the weight resting on your sitting bones and through the balance points under your feet (see pages 136–37).
- Lengthen up through the spine while, at the same time, drawing your shoulder blades downward.
- Engage the centering muscles to help create an overall sense of lightness within your body.

Adopt this position as far as possible for all of your seated activities. Avoid sitting in soft, low chairs for long periods of time. They may seem restful at the time but gradually they can do a great deal of harm to your back. Also ensure that your office chair is properly adjusted for your height, otherwise your back will be placed under extra stress and this will cause it to be strained.

SEATED SIDE STRETCHES

The side stretches shown here engage the deep muscles in the sides of the body, and so contribute to the overall strength of the torso while also encouraging greater mobility. One of the key factors to effective side stretches is to use your centering muscles to maintain a sense of lifting and lengthening as well as bending or rotating. This keeps the spine well supported through the movement and prevents compression of the intervertebral disks. The other vital element is the maintenance of a stable pelvis to provide a firm anchor for the stretches. Working in the sitting position helps to immobilize the pelvis, but you will also have to use the lower abdominal muscles.

Side stretch

1 *Sit toward the edge of a firm chair with your knees hip-width apart. Slide your shoulder blades down your back, engage your centering muscles and lengthen up through the spine. Place your hands behind your head.*

2 *On an out-breath stretch over to one side. Control the movement with your centering muscles. Come back to the center on an in-breath. Repeat to the other side. Complete six repetitions.*

Seated rotation

1 *Adopt the same starting position as for the side stretch.*

Head and neck follow the movement

Elbows wide apart in line with shoulders

Centering muscles control the movement

2 *On an out-breath, engage the centering muscles and rotate your body to one side. Keep the pelvis completely still and facing forward. Breathe in to return to center. Repeat on the other side. Repeat six times.*

195

Working the Sides of the Legs

Cushion support
Use a cushion to support your upper leg to ensure alignment of the pelvis in the inner thigh lift.

There are not many everyday activities that effectively strengthen and tone the inner and outer muscles of the thigh and hip. However these are important muscles for the maintenance of proper alignment of the legs and pelvis. They also contribute to the effectiveness of the leg movements.

The success of the exercises in this group depend on the precise alignment of the spine in the side position. When you first start learning these exercises it is useful to align your sacrum and back against a wall so that you can be sure that you have adopted the right position. Having successfully established this position, you need to keep your

centering muscles strongly engaged throughout the sequence in order to maintain it. The need for such control is the reason why these exercises are classed as progression exercises; you need to have developed a good level of stability in the torso before you can perform them successfully.

From waist to thigh

The outer thigh exercises that form the first part of this set not only work the muscles along the outside of the thigh from the hip to the knee, but also strengthen and tone the waist, buttocks (gluteals), and deep muscles that control the hip joint. When you are performing the exercises you will soon become aware of the muscles being worked. But don't allow the effort to create tension in your body. Keep the following body-awareness pointers in mind:

- Maintain a sense of lengthening from your neck all the way through to the heel of the working leg.
- Visualize the movement originating in the waist and keep your waist "long" so that your pelvis remains stable as you move your leg.

Working the inner thigh

The adductor muscles of the inner thigh are the focus of the next exercise you will be shown. But it is important to remember to support the entire action by using your centering muscles; this will ensure that the effort remains located in the intended area. Keep in mind that, although you are lying down, you are not supposed to be resting. Some beginners find it difficult to maintain a stable position while performing this exercise since there can be a tendency for the hip to tip forward. It may therefore be helpful to use a firm pillow or folded towel to support the upper leg while doing this exercise.

SIDE LEG LIFTS

Before you begin these exercises you should spend some time checking your alignment in the side position. As a newcomer to this part of the program, it is best to lie against a wall to help you establish the correct position. When you have become accustomed to the exercise, you will probably find that you can adopt the position without the help of the wall. Make sure you are comfortable lying on your side and use a layer of padding under your hip if you need the extra support. Complete six repetitions of each exercise on one side and then turn and repeat on the other.

Mat for extra support

Starting position

Lie on your side with your underneath arm stretched out above your head and place your other hand in front of your body to prevent yourself from tipping forward. Bend your knees at right angles and then check that your top foot is directly above the lower one and that your knees, hips, and shoulders are similarly stacked. You can use a mat for extra support.

Outer thigh lifts

1 *Straighten your top leg so that the foot is a short distance from the floor. Flex your foot and angle it downward. Breathe in.*

2 *On the out-breath, raise your top leg a little further. Keep your body stable. Breathe in and lower your leg.*

Inner thigh lifts

1 *Extend the lower leg and bend the upper leg at right angles. Support the upper knee with a plump cushion to prevent the hips from rolling forward.*

2 *Breathe in. On the out-breath engage the centering muscles and lift the lower leg a couple of inches. Lower on the out-breath, maintaining the stability of the torso and pelvis as you do so.*

Releasing Tension in the Chest

Supporting the neck & head
*For the chest opening exercise it is important
to keep the head and neck in alignment with
the spine. A firm cushion under the head
will help you achieve this.*

When under threat our natural instinct is to close in around the chest and abdomen. This is to protect the vital organs from injury in case of attack. We carry this instinctive reaction into our daily life—even in a modern urban society. As we deal with the stress and worry that is part of a normal busy routine, muscle tension and a sense of restriction in the chest can build up insidiously as we sit hunched over a desk or cramped in a car, for example, for hours on end. Breathing becomes shallow and the muscles in the shoulders and chest tighten. Ineffective breathing only adds to the physical tension and increases fatigue and irritability. Often we are unaware of this happening. It is only when we consciously work to release these tensions through gentle stretches such as the chest opening exercise on the following pages that we realize the damaging effect of this physical manifestation of stress.

Releasing muscle tension

The chest opening exercise also helps to relax hard-worked muscles after a serious exercise session, helping you to avoid possible stiffness and feel both reinvigorated and at peace.

Approach this exercise in a leisurely fashion, and allow yourself to relish the sense of release that it will bring. Focus on the sensation of "openness" that the movement induces. Try to visualize the muscles of the upper chest slowly stretching out, encouraged by your steady breathing and relaxation of the shoulders.

Progressing gradually

As with all Pilates exercise, it is your approach to the movement that is important, not the final position you achieve. In this case you should focus on getting your starting position correct and maintaining the alignment of the pelvis and knees. Although you are aiming to reach the floor with your top arm as you lift it to the other side of your body, if you are stiff you may not manage this at first. However, you will still be gaining the full benefit of a valuable stretch, providing you perform the exercise precisely. In a few weeks you will find that increased mobility in your spine and shoulders will permit you to stretch further.

CHEST OPENING

For this exercise you need to position yourself carefully before you start so that your head, neck, and spine are in alignment. Your knees should be bent so as to create a right angle between your torso and thighs and between the thighs and lower legs. Your arms should also be stretched out in front at right angles to the body. Throughout the movement your aim should be to keep your pelvis and legs completely stable. All movement should be focused in your upper body.

1 *Lie on your side with your head resting on a cushion and your knees bent at right angles to your body. Make sure that your hips are aligned vertically and your knees and feet are together. Stretch your arms out in front, fingers together.*

Knees together

Elbows soft

2 Breathe in and engage your centering muscles to stabilize your pelvis. Lift your top arm slowly in an arc over your body. Follow its movement with your head. Keep your gaze on your hand. Keep your arm relaxed and your elbow soft.

3 Take your arm as far toward the floor as is comfortable. You will know you have reached your limit if you feel your hips or knees shifting out of alignment. Return to the starting position on an out-breath. Repeat five times.

Pelvis
stable

Head and eyes
follow movement

Wrapping Up

Record-keeping

Write down difficulties you have experienced and overcome as well as the benefits you notice from your training.

As you finish each of your Pilates sessions you need to wind down without losing the sense of energy that you have generated during the course of your workout. You therefore need to provide your body with a sense of balance and harmony that integrates the beneficial effects on different parts of the body of the various exercises you have performed. Moreover, the final exercise that you perform will have a bearing on the feelings that you take away from your workout. A complex exercise, which you may have some difficulty mastering, could leave you

with a sense of dissatisfaction or even failure. So it is important to choose an accessible exercise that leaves you in a state of physical harmony and with positive emotions. You should also be aiming to relax your whole body before you finish, which is an important part of the last exercise.

The final stretch
The full body stretch on the following pages provides an ideal close to your exercise session. It allows active relaxation for the whole body—from head to toe. You will by now have a full appreciation of the degree of active engagement that you need to incorporate into any stretching exercise, and this one is no different. But this effort is always balanced by a wonderful sense of release and relaxation when the stretch is complete. For variety you may sometimes choose to end your Pilates session with a different closing exercise. The chest opening stretch on page 202 and the roll downs foundation exercise on page 130 are excellent alternatives. Be sure to perform whichever exercise you choose slowly and with care.

When you have repeated your final stretch a few times, you should allow yourself time for relaxation as you gradually ready your mind and body for a return to your regular activities.

Self-assessment

Once an exercise session has finished, it is easy to forget the detail of what exercises you performed, how many repetitions, how easy or difficult you found them, and whether you had any particular problems. Try keeping a diary of your progress that you can update after each session. This information will be useful in planning your ongoing Pilates program. It will help you to pinpoint which exercises you need to work on and which aspects are causing you problems. If you are working under the guidance of a Pilates teacher, these notes can provide valuable feedback for discussion at your next lesson.

FULL BODY STRETCH

Use this exercise as your final wind-down after your Pilates session. It can also be used as an instant relaxer and reenergizer anytime you need to release physical and mental tension: for example, after returning home from work or after any other tiring activity. Remember that the more energy you put into the stretch, the greater the sense of relaxation there will be when you release it. Be sure to check your alignment in the supine position before you start (see pages 48–49). When you have finished, you should be careful how you get up. Sudden movements will disrupt the feeling of tranquility you have acquired and may also make you feel dizzy.

Lie on your back in the neutral position with your legs straight. Extend your arms over your head. On an out-breath, stretch out from your toes to your fingertips. Keep your shoulders relaxed and away from your ears. Repeat this movement up to five times and then relax (see box).

Hands and fingers
extended

Shoulders down

Waist
lengthened

Relaxation

After the full body stretch, allow yourself a few minutes' relaxation before getting up. Choose a comfortable lying-down position on your back or side. If necessary, use cushions to support yourself in a strain-free position. Focus on your breathing and the sensation of your weight sinking into the floor.

Knees extended, but soft

Feet pointed, toes relaxed

Working with Weights

Choosing weights
You can buy weights from a sports supplier or improvise with household items such as bags of rice or sugar.

Using weights, whether they are handheld or strapped to the wrists or ankles, will increase the workload of any exercise involving arm or leg movements. The relevent muscles have to work harder to overcome the resistance created by the weight and therefore will eventually become stronger and more toned than they would have been if no weights had been used. There is also a general relationship between the lifting of heavy weights and the development of muscle bulk. However, that is not the aim of using weights in Pilates exercise, in which the relatively light weights used and the careful balance of the exercises means that the added muscle bulk is minimal.

Strong muscles, strong bones

Over the past few decades, medical research into the causes of the common bone-thinning condition osteoporosis has indicated a strong correlation between the amount of weight-bearing exercise undertaken during adult life and bone density. It is clear that those who regularly get such exercise have a much lower risk of osteoporosis than those who don't. This is especially important for women, who are far more susceptible to loss of bone mass after menopause than men of a similar age. All Pilates exercise is helpful for maintaining bone density, but adding weights increases this benefit.

When to add weights

Do not feel pressured to add weights to your practice. You can exercise effectively against the resistance of your own body weight and with regular practice you will continue to progress. But if you do want to add weights you need to observe some guidelines. There is no point in adding weights until you have mastered the basic technique for any exercise and have built up the necessary level of strength. Be sure that you can perform the recommended number of repetitions of the exercise, while maintaining complete muscular control (with stable, neutral pelvis, ribs drawn in, shoulder blades down the back, and all centering muscles engaged) before attempting to make this transition. If you are working with a Pilates teacher, ask their advice on the right time for you to start using weights.

Which weights to use

Always start with the lightest weights. For your first practices with handheld weights, experiment with cans of food or packages of rice or sugar, for example, weighing 8–17 ounces (250–500 grams). If you make progress with these starter weights, you may wish to graduate to something a little heavier. If you want to buy weights, choose dumbbells and/or strap-on ankle weights of no more than 2 pounds (0.9 kilograms) for the first few months of weight practice.

ADDING WEIGHTS
Holding a weight in each hand increases the workload of all exercises involving arm movements. Depending on the exercise, this can further strengthen and tone your arm, shoulder, chest, and back muscles. Adding weights to your ankles increases the workload in exercises that involve leg movements. This can provide an extra challenge to your leg, hip, buttock, and lower abdominal muscles.

SHOULDER WORK —
ARMS TOGETHER

ARM WORK

SHOULDER WORK—
ALTERNATING ARMS

OUTER LEG WORK

INNER LEG WORK

Achieving Integration

The whole body

Your aim is to develop a sense of all parts of your body functioning together as an integrated whole.

This is a book for newcomers to Pilates. Even when you've read all the material it contains, assimilated the information and instructions, and tried all the exercises, you will still be a relative novice. Reeducating your body away from its previous bad habits and continually reinforcing the healthier ways of moving is a lifetime project. The learning curve is steep when you first start and flattens as you build on the increasingly familiar

principles of Pilates. But as you progress you will begin to appreciate that there are new levels to which you can take your understanding and physical abilities.

What is integration?

The word integration, when used in a Pilates context, generally refers to the balanced development of all the muscles in the body. The strengthening of one group of muscles should never be allowed to distort the functioning of a less developed muscle group. This integration can be achieved only through years of balanced practice. You need determination and dedication to commit yourself to a program of exercises that includes many movements you find difficult and exhausting as well as those you find easy and enjoyable.

Continuous movement

The idea of integration can also be applied to the way you practice your Pilates exercises. As a novice, you will have been focusing all your attention on executing the individual exercises to the best of your ability. And this is the way it should be. However, once you are thoroughly familiar with a basic selection

of exercises and can perform them
all fluently, you may wish to consider
integrating them into a single continuous
movement, in which one exercise flows
into the next like a dance. This kind of
practice enables you to develop further
the essential Pilates principles of fluidity
and coordination and bring into your
exercise program an element of creativity
as you devise your own combinations of
movements.

When you work in this way, your
exercise routine will be far removed from
the tedious drudgery that some people
consider it to be. You will find that it is in
fact a time for self-expression and physical
harmony and will look forward to your
exercise session each day. See the
sequence on the following pages as an
example of how to advance from your
basic exercises.

PILATES AS DANCE

The series of exercises on this page gives an example of how you can link individual exercises to form a continuous dancelike movement. Use your imagination to devise your own dances from combinations of exercises that you are confident in performing well. Be careful to ensure that transitions between exercises are performed smoothly and without jerkiness. Remember that control and precision in your movements remain your governing principles.

6

7

8

9

10

11

12

GLOSSARY

Abdominals The muscles that surround and support the area from the ribcage to the pubic bone. They control the movement of the torso and are the basis of the girdle of strength.

Body awareness Refers to sensitivity to the effects on your body of different physical actions. This includes awareness of your posture and alignment and which muscles are being utilized in each movement.

Centering muscles Used to describe the muscles that support the center of the body. These include the abdominal muscles, pelvic floor, latissimus dorsi, and gluteals.

Contrology The name Joseph Pilates gave to his system of body-conditioning exercises.

Engagement A muscle is said to be engaged when it is active and contracted during a movement. In Pilates-based exercise you learn to engage muscles without bringing tension or stiffness into the action.

Girdle of strength Describes the muscles that support the center of the body.

Gluteals, gluteus maximus The large muscles of the buttocks, attached to the sacrum and the upper part of the femur.

Hamstrings The muscles at the back of the thigh that contract to bend the knee.

Hip width The distance between an individual's hip joints, often used as a measure for the placement of the feet in Pilates exercise because it ensures correct parallel alignment of the hips, knees, and ankles.

Latissimus dorsi The muscles that extend from the shoulder blades to the top of the pelvis. Commonly known as the lats, they stabilize the shoulder blades and provide postural support.

Lumbar curve The natural concave curve in the spine at the waist.

Mobilization The restoration or enhancement of the range of movement in a joint. Pilates aims to mobilize joints such as the hips, shoulders, and intervertebral joints to give stress-free movement.

Navel to spine The action of drawing in the abdominal muscles on exhalation, which promotes hollowing or "scooping" of the tummy. This action engages the deep muscles within the abdomen that support the spine and ensures that all the centering muscles are working together correctly to produce a strong and streamlined torso.

Neutral pelvis, neutral spine The position of the pelvis that creates the correct curves in the spine. If the top of the pelvis tips forward, the lumbar curve is exaggerated. If it tips back, the lumbar curve is flattened. In most Pilates exercises, the pelvis and spine need to be held in the neutral position.

Obliques The muscles that stretch diagonally around the sides of the body and meet in the front of the abdomen. These are important centering muscles that govern the twisting movements of the torso.

Pelvic floor The hammock of muscles that run from the pubic bone to the sacrum. These provide support for the pelvic organs and also contribute to posture and alignment.

Pelvis The bony basin that protects the vital lower abdominal organs. It is attached to the lower part of the spine and is the anchoring point for the hip joints.

Powerhouse A term used by Joseph Pilates for the girdle of strength.

Prone Describes the position in which you are lying, face downward, on the abdomen.

Quadriceps The large muscles at the front of the thigh, also known as the quads, that contract to lift the thigh and extend the knee joint.

Rectus abdominus The vertical sheet of muscle at the front of the abdomen. Contraction of this centering muscle flexes the body forward.

Sacrum The large flat bone near the base of the spine that is joined to the back of the pelvis.

Scoop A term used by some Pilates teachers to describe the hollowing effect of drawing the navel to the spine.

Supine Lying face up on your back.

Thoracic breathing Also known as rib breathing, this method of expanding the ribcage out to the sides to draw in air, rather than expanding the abdomen, is used in most Pilates exercises. In this method the ribcage contracts on the out-breath, allowing effective engagement of the centering muscles during any movement requiring effort.

Transversus abdominus The transversus muscles of the abdomen wrap around the center of the body and provide support for the abdominal organs.

Trapezius The diamond-shaped muscle that extends from the neck outward to each shoulder and down between the shoulder blades. This muscle tends to contract and remain bunched and tense when we are under stress. This distorts the position of the shoulders and in turn can lead to headaches and a variety of postural problems.

FURTHER READING

Benson, Herbert M.D. *The Relaxation Response.* Avon Books, 2000.

Bussell, Darcey. *Pilates for Life.* Michael Joseph, 2005.

Isacowitz, Rael. *Pilates.* Human Kinetics Europe Ltd;. 2014.

Isacowitz, Rael, and Karen Clippinger. *Pilates Anatomy.* Human Kinetics Publishers, 2011.

Lawrence, Debbie. *Pilates Method: An Integrative Approach to Teaching.* A&C Black, 2008.

Pilates, Joseph H. *Your Health: A Corrective System of Exercising That Revolutionizes the Entire Field of Physical Education.* Presentation Dynamics Inc., 1998.

Pilates, Joseph H., and William J. Miller. *Pilates' Return to Life Through Contrology.* Presentation Dynamics Inc., 1998.

Robinson, Lynn, Lisa Bradshaw, and Nathan Gardner. *The Pilates Bible.* Kyle Cathie, 2010.

Robinson, Lynn, Helge Fisher, and Paul Massey. *The Body Control Pilates Back Book.* Pan Books, 2002.

Robinson, Lynn, and Gordon Thomson. *The Official Body Control Pilates Manual.* Macmillan, 2000.

Robinson, Lynn, Carmela Trappa, and Jenny Hawke. *Pilates for Life: How to Improve Strength, Flexibility and Healthy Over 40.* Kyle Books, 2014.

Siler, Brooke. *The Pilates Body.* Michael Joseph, 2000.

Ungaro, Alycea. *Pilates Body in Motion.* Dorling Kindersley, 2016.

USEFUL ADDRESSES

The Australian Pilates Method Association
www.australianpilates.asn.au
A nonprfofit organization aimed at promoting and teaching the benefits of the Pilates method to a diverse range of the population.

Balanced Body
www.pilates.com
A general information website

The Body Control Pilates Association
www.bodycontrolpilates.com
Home to the UK's largest Pilates facility, based in London, with studios offering matwork classes and training.

Moretti Studio
www.pilates-montreal.com
Information on the Montreal studio directed and instructed by Daniela Moretti.

The Pilates Center
www.thepilatescenter.com
Colorado-based studio offering private lessons, group classes, and a teacher training program.

Pilates Method Alliance
www.pilatesmethodalliance.org
Home of the professional association and certifying agency for Pilates teachers.

The Pilates Foundation
www.pilatesfoundation.com
The UK's first Pilates Teachers' Association, providing information on Pilates classes and teachers in your area.

The Pilates Studio
www.pilates-studio.com
Information on the New York Pilates Studio Teacher Certification Program.

The Pilates Studio® of Los Angeles
www.pilatestherapy.com
Information on the Los Angeles Pilates and Physical Therapy Fitness Center, offering therapy, exercise, and pilates teacher certification.

Pilatesstyle
www.pilatesstyle.com
A magazine with useful information on Pilates exercises and studios.

INDEX

ACKNOWLEDGMENTS

Every effort has been made to trace copyright holders and obtain permission. The publishers apologise for any omissions and would be pleased to make any necessary changes at subsequent printings.

PICTURE ACKNOWLEDGMENTS

Getty/4x6: 14–15; BJI / Lane Oatey: 117; BLOOM image: 193; Milena Boniek: 181; Angela Coppola: 145; blwilliamsphoto: 67; Dominique Douieb: 197; Johnny Greig: 45; Image Source: 61, 189; PhotoAlto: 179; PhotoAlto/Frederic Cirou: 129; PhotoAlto/Sandro Di Carlo Darsa: 89; I C Rapoport / Contributor: 13; John Slater: 47; Ben Welsh: 2; Westend61: 169. **iStock**/andresr: 201; andresrimaging: 157; annebaek: 68; binabina: 31T; DenisovDmitry: 9, 218; Jim Jurica: 77; Stigur Karlsson: 33; Neustockimages: 64, 219; skynesher: 71, 209. **Shutterstock**/Guryanov Andrey: 97; Alexander Y: 213; Alexlukin: 204; carlo dapino: 101; Dean Drobot: 8; Djurdjevic: 5; fizkes: 6T, 44, 66, 69, 125, 141, 205; Vladimir Gjorgiev: 137; glebTv: 85; gosphotodesign: 28; Iasha: 161; Anna Jurkovska: 35; Karramba Production: 143; Elena Kharichkina: 153; Elizabeta Lexa: 4, 224; maradon 333: 212; Michael Pettigrew: 30T; mykeyruna: 29; Nicolesa: 11; ra2studio: 12, 185; Summersky: 140; Syda Productions: 65; Olena Yakobchuk: 165.